FAMILY MEDICINE POCKET GUIDE

Rural Edition

DR. MOHAMED ELGENDY
LMCC, CCFP CANADA

DISCLAIMER

This pocket guide was developed with the assistance of advanced AI tools to streamline content generation. Every chapter has been thoroughly reviewed, edited, and authenticated by Dr. Mohamed Elgendy, LMCC, CCFP (Canada), ensuring accuracy, credibility, and clinical authenticity. The result is a modern, innovative reference that blends the efficiency of AI with the rigor of professional medical expertise.

This booklet summarizes common family medicine and rural primary-care approaches using open-access guidance only; no proprietary or subscription-based content is reproduced. Clinical descriptions (including assessments, investigations, and treatments) are abbreviated for educational purposes and exam preparation. They are not intended as complete protocols or substitutes for independent clinical judgment.

Management should always be performed within the clinician's scope of training, local regulations, and available resources, with appropriate patient consent, monitoring, and safety measures. Escalate care promptly when red flags arise (e.g., airway compromise, hemodynamic instability, severe infection, suspected surgical emergency, or complex multi-morbidity) or when the situation exceeds your competence or resources.

Always confirm current local and national guidelines, product monographs/labels, and institutional pathways before application. Verify patient-specific contraindications, comorbidities, and drug interactions. Clinical responsibility remains with the treating clinician.

DEDICATION

This booklet is dedicated to the patients in rural and remote communities—whose resilience, trust, and courage guide every decision; to the clinicians, nurses, medics, and staff who deliver essential procedures with skill, compassion, and ingenuity despite distance and limited resources; to mentors and colleagues who share knowledge openly so care can remain safe and evidence-informed; and to my family, whose steady support makes this work possible. May this concise, open-access procedure booklet serve them all.

— *Dr. Mohamed Elgendy*

ABOUT THE AUTHIOR

Dr. Mohamed Elgendy is a licensed Canadian physician with the Licentiate of the Medical Council of Canada (LMCC) and Certification in Family Medicine (CCFP) from the College of Family Physicians of Canada.

He has extensive hands-on experience as both a rural emergency physician and family doctor, currently practicing in Saskatchewan, Canada. With a deep commitment to improving emergency and acute care in underserved communities, Dr. Elgendy focuses on practical, evidence-based emergency medicine adapted to the realities of rural practice.

His work bridges the gap between academic guidelines and frontline clinical realities, offering accessible, concise resources to help clinicians make confident, lifesaving decisions in resource-limited settings.

PROCEDURES INDEX — CATEGORIZED

CARDIOVASCULAR

SECONDARY HYPERTENSION — FAMILY MEDICINE OFFICE

OVERVIEW & "DON'T MISS"

1. ≈5–10% of hypertension has a specific, potentially reversible cause. Consider when onset <30 or >55 yrs, abrupt/worsening BP, resistant HTN (≥3 drugs incl. diuretic), severe/accelerated HTN, or suggestive clinical clues.

2. Common causes: renal parenchymal disease; renovascular disease (atherosclerotic RAS, fibromuscular dysplasia); primary aldosteronism; obstructive sleep apnea (OSA); thyroid/parathyroid disease; Cushing syndrome; pheochromocytoma; coarctation of aorta (younger); medication/ substance-induced.

3. DON'T MISS: hypertensive emergency (encephalopathy, ACS, AHF, stroke, AKI); pheochromocytoma crisis; flash pulmonary edema from bilateral RAS; aortic dissection; preeclampsia/ HELLP.

HISTORY & EXAM

1. Onset/timeline; prior BPs; adherence; family history of early HTN/stroke; sleep/snoring/daytime somnolence; episodic headaches, palpitations, diaphoresis (pheo); muscle weakness/cramps/polydipsia/polyuria (hypokalemia/PA).
2. Medication/substances: NSAIDs, oral contraceptives, decongestants, steroids, calcineurin inhibitors, erythropoietin, stimulants/cocaine/amphetamines, licorice/herbals, alcohol.
3. Comorbid: CKD, DM, obesity, OSA, thyroid disease, pregnancy plans.
4. Exam: accurate BP (both arms; consider ABPM/HBPM), BMI/neck circumference, abdominal bruits, radio-femoral delay/arm-leg BP gradient (coarctation), fundi (hypertensive retinopathy), thyroid, edema, signs of Cushing, pulses/perfusion.

DIFFERENTIAL DIAGNOSIS (TOP 5)

1. Primary (essential) hypertension with poor technique/adherence ('pseudo-resistance').
2. Renal parenchymal disease (CKD).
3. Primary aldosteronism (with or without hypokalemia).
4. Renovascular hypertension (RAS/FMD).
5. Obstructive sleep apnea–related hypertension.

INVESTIGATIONS (POC/LABS/IMAGING)

1. Initial for all HTN: BMP (Cr/eGFR, K$^+$), fasting glucose/

A1C, fasting lipids, urinalysis ± ACR, TSH, ECG; pregnancy test if applicable.

2. If resistant HTN or clues → targeted tests:

3. Primary aldosteronism (PA): morning seated aldosterone-renin ratio (ARR). Correct hypokalemia; liberalize sodium for a few days. Hold MRAs (spironolactone/eplerenone) 4–6 wks if feasible; minimize β-blockers/central α-2 agonists that ↓ renin; ACEi/ARB/diuretics can alter results — interpret with lab. Positive screen (e.g., ARR elevated with plasma aldosterone typically >10 ng/dL [~275 pmol/L]) → confirmatory testing (saline/oral salt load) and adrenal imaging ± AVS.

4. Renovascular disease: renal function/ACR; duplex renal artery Doppler (operator-dependent). CTA/MRA for high suspicion (bilateral RAS, solitary kidney with RAS, flash pulmonary edema, rise in Cr after ACEi/ARB).

5. Pheochromocytoma: plasma free metanephrines or 24-h urinary fractionated metanephrines (draw supine after rest if possible).

6. Cushing syndrome: 1-mg overnight dexamethasone suppression test OR late-night salivary cortisol (×2) OR 24-h urinary free cortisol (×2).

7. OSA: STOP-Bang screen → home sleep apnea test/polysomnography if positive.

8. Coarctation (younger): arm-leg BP difference, diminished femoral pulses; echo/CT/MR angiography.

9. Thyroid/parathyroid: TSH (already above); calcium for hyperparathyroidism if hypercalcemia symptoms.

MANAGEMENT (NON-PHARM → MEDS → PROCEDURES)

A. NON-PHARMACOLOGIC

1. DASH diet, sodium <1500–2000 mg/day, weight loss (5–10%), aerobic/resistance exercise, alcohol moderation, stop tobacco, sleep hygiene and CPAP adherence when OSA.
2. Home BP monitoring/ABPM to confirm control; medication adherence supports (once-daily combos, blister packs).

B. MEDICATIONS (TREAT CAUSE + CONTROL BP; INDIVIDUALIZE)

1. Renal parenchymal disease: ACEi/ARB first-line (proteinuric CKD); add thiazide-like (chlorthalidone) if GFR >30 or loop if GFR lower; add DHP-CCB; monitor K^+/Cr.
2. Primary aldosteronism: mineralocorticoid receptor antagonists (spironolactone 12.5–50 mg/day or eplerenone 25–50 mg BID). Unilateral aldosterone-producing adenoma → adrenalectomy after AVS confirmation where appropriate.
3. Renovascular HTN: optimal medical therapy (ACEi/ARB, statin, antiplatelet if indicated). Revascularization for select high-risk phenotypes (recurrent flash

pulmonary edema, refractory HTN, progressive renal dysfunction with bilateral RAS or solitary kidney).

4. Pheochromocytoma: α-blockade FIRST (phenoxybenzamine or doxazosin) ± high-salt diet/ volume expansion, then β-blocker if needed; definitive surgical resection; endocrine + surgical referral.

5. Cushing syndrome: treat underlying source (pituitary/ adrenal/ectopic); endocrine referral.

6. OSA: CPAP + weight loss improves BP and CV risk.

7. Coarctation: cardiology referral for repair (surgery/ stent).

8. Medication/substance-induced: stop/replace offending agents (NSAIDs, OCPs with estrogen, decongestants, stimulants, calcineurin inhibitors, licorice). Consider progestin-only/IUD for contraception.

C. PROCEDURES

1. Ambulatory BP monitoring orders; arrange imaging (renal Doppler/CTA/MRA), sleep studies, endocrine dynamic tests; refer for AVS, revascularization, or surgery when indicated.

DISPOSITION (DISCHARGE/OBSERVE/ TRANSFER) & RETURN PRECAUTIONS

1. Discharge: stable BP plan, lifestyle counselling, labs ordered (K^+/Cr 1–2 weeks after ACEi/ARB/MRA changes), and referrals placed; follow-up 2–4 weeks for resistant HTN.

2. Urgent/Same-day: hypertensive urgency with symptoms, suspected pheo crisis (severe headache, diaphoresis, pallor, tachycardia), acute rise in Cr with ACEi/ARB in bilateral RAS/solitary kidney, or pregnancy with severe HTN $\rightarrow$ ED.

3. Return immediately: chest pain, neuro deficits, severe dyspnea, syncope, visual loss, or BP $\geq$180/120 with symptoms.

PEARLS & PITFALLS

1. Screen for primary aldosteronism in resistant HTN or HTN with spontaneous/diuretic-induced hypokalemia (even if K^+ normal).

2. Correct hypokalemia before ARR; know drug effects on renin/aldosterone and coordinate safe temporary adjustments.

3. Young woman with HTN + abdominal bruit $\rightarrow$ think fibromuscular dysplasia; consider renal artery imaging.

4. Avoid β-blocker before α-blocker in pheochromocytoma (risk of unopposed α and crisis).

5. Confirm elevated office BP with HBPM/ABPM to avoid overtreatment of white-coat HTN.

REFERENCES

1. NICE Guideline NG136. Hypertension in adults: diagnosis and management (open). nice.org.uk

2. Endocrine Society Clinical Practice Guideline (2016). Primary Aldosteronism: Case Detection, Diagnosis,

and Treatment — open summary. endocrine.org / journals summaries

3. American Heart Association (AHA) Scientific Statements on Secondary Hypertension and Resistant Hypertension — open summaries. heart.org

4. European Society of Cardiology/European Society of Hypertension (ESC/ESH) Guidelines — key points open access. escardio.org

5. AAFP. Diagnosis of Secondary Hypertension: An Age-Based Approach; Resistant Hypertension — open articles. aafp.org

6. BC Guidelines. Hypertension — Provincial algorithm with secondary causes and work-up (public). bcguidelines.gov.bc.ca

7. Radiology/Imaging: ACR Appropriateness Criteria® — Renovascular Hypertension (public). acsearch.acr.org

ESSENTIAL (PRIMARY) HYPERTENSION

OVERVIEW & "DON'T MISS"

1. Very common, often asymptomatic; major driver of stroke, MI, HF, CKD.

2. Confirm with out-of-office BP (ABPM/HBPM) before labeling and treating when feasible.

3. DON'T MISS hypertensive emergency: BP ≥180/120 mmHg WITH acute end-organ symptoms (chest pain, neuro deficits, vision loss, acute dyspnea, AKI, eclampsia, aortic pain). Immediate ED transfer.

4. Consider secondary causes when severe/resistant, abrupt onset, age <30, hypokalemia, renal bruit, or acute kidney function drop.

HISTORY & EXAM

1. History: duration; home BP; meds (NSAIDs, decongestants, OCPs, steroids, stimulants, calcineurin inhibitors), alcohol, substances (cocaine/amphetamines), sleep apnea, kidney disease, thyroid; CVD/CKD/DM; pregnancy status; symptoms of end-organ damage.

2. Exam: standardized seated BP (validated device,

correct cuff, both arms), BMI/waist; pulses/bruits; fundoscopic exam; thyroid; cardiac/pulmonary; edema; signs suggesting secondary HTN.

DIFFERENTIAL DIAGNOSIS (TOP 5)

1. White-coat hypertension (elevated office, normal ABPM/HBPM).
2. Masked hypertension (normal office, elevated ABPM/HBPM).
3. Secondary hypertension: renal parenchymal & renovascular disease, primary aldosteronism, OSA, endocrine (thyroid, pheochromocytoma, Cushing).
4. Medication/substance-induced (NSAIDs, OCPs, steroids, stimulants, alcohol, cocaine).
5. Transient BP elevation from pain/anxiety/illness — not persistent HTN.

INVESTIGATIONS (POC/LABS/IMAGING)

1. POC/Clinic: repeated standardized office BP; ABPM (preferred) or 7-day HBPM to confirm diagnosis when feasible; ECG baseline.
2. Labs (baseline): CBC, electrolytes, creatinine/eGFR, fasting lipids, A1C or fasting glucose, TSH (if clinically indicated), urinalysis ± albumin-creatinine ratio.
3. Consider: renin/aldosterone if hypokalemia or resistant HTN; sleep apnea screening; pregnancy test when applicable.
4. Imaging: renal ultrasound if abnormal renal function/

UA; renal artery imaging if high suspicion of renovascular disease; echocardiogram if symptoms/ signs of LV dysfunction.

MANAGEMENT (NON-PHARM → MEDS → PROCEDURES)

A. NON-PHARMACOLOGIC (FIRST-LINE FOR ALL)

1. Weight loss (5–10% body weight), aerobic activity 150–300 min/week; muscle-strengthening 2+ days/ week.
2. DASH-style eating pattern; sodium intake reduction (≈ <2 g/day sodium); increase potassium in diet if not contraindicated.
3. Limit alcohol; stop smoking; optimize sleep and treat OSA; stress management; home BP monitoring with a validated device.

B. PHARMACOLOGIC (ADULT DOSING EXAMPLES; INDIVIDUALIZE)

1. Start meds if BP ≥140/90 mmHg, or if SBP 130–139 mmHg with high CVD risk (established CVD, diabetes, CKD, 10-yr FRS ≥20%, or age ≥75). Target: systolic BP <130 mmHg if tolerated.
2. Initial therapy: low-dose combination (prefer single-pill) using TWO of: (1) ACE inhibitor or ARB, (2) thiazide-like diuretic (e.g., chlorthalidone 12.5–25 mg daily or indapamide 1.25–2.5 mg daily), (3) long-acting dihydropyridine CCB (e.g., amlodipine 5–10 mg daily).

3. ACEi examples: ramipril 2.5–10 mg daily; perindopril 4–8 mg daily. ARB examples: losartan 50–100 mg daily; valsartan 80–320 mg daily.

4. If not at target: uptitrate, then add third agent. Resistant HTN: add spironolactone 12.5–25 mg daily (monitor K+/creatinine).

5. Beta-blocker when compelling indications (e.g., ischemic heart disease, HFrEF, arrhythmia) — not first-line for uncomplicated HTN.

6. Avoid ACEi + ARB combination; review teratogenicity (avoid ACEi/ARB in pregnancy); check electrolytes/ creatinine 1–2 weeks after starting/increasing ACEi/ ARB or diuretic.

C. PROCEDURES

1. None routinely in primary care for essential HTN; focus on lifestyle + pharmacotherapy and investigation of secondary causes when indicated.

DISPOSITION (DISCHARGE/OBSERVE/ TRANSFER) & RETURN PRECAUTIONS

1. Discharge (most): asymptomatic, no end-organ findings → begin/adjust therapy, education, arrange follow-up in 2–4 weeks with home BP log.

2. Observe same-day or urgent follow-up: very high BP (e.g., ≥180/110) without symptoms, new abnormal labs, or diagnostic uncertainty.

3. Transfer to ED: suspected hypertensive EMERGENCY

(acute neuro deficits, chest pain/ACS, acute HF/
pulmonary edema, vision loss, aortic pain, eclampsia,
AKI).

4. Return immediately if red-flag symptoms above;
   otherwise return if home SBP persistently ≥160 or DBP
   ≥100 despite adherence.

PEARLS & PITFALLS

1. Always confirm diagnosis with ABPM/HBPM when
   feasible; masked/white-coat patterns are common.

2. Use validated devices and proper cuff size; measure
   both arms initially; watch for orthostatic hypotension in
   older/frail patients.

3. Prioritize single-pill combinations to improve
   adherence; reassess every 1–3 months until at target.

4. Check for secondary causes and BP-raising meds
   (NSAIDs, decongestants, stimulants).

5. Document shared decision-making and safety-netting.

REFERENCES

1. Hypertension Canada. 2025 Primary Care Guideline.
   CMAJ (Supplement). Public PDF: hypertension.ca
   (Accessed 2025-08-16).

2. BC Guidelines. Hypertension — Diagnosis &
   Management (updated 2024). Public guideline:
   bcguidelines.gov.bc.ca (Accessed 2025-08-16).

3. NICE Guideline NG136. Hypertension in adults:
   diagnosis and management (last reviewed 2024).

Public: nice.org.uk (Accessed 2025-08-16).

4. USPSTF. Hypertension in Adults: Screening (2021 Recommendation). Public: uspreventiveservicestaskforce.org (Accessed 2025-08-16).

5. WHO. Guideline for the pharmacological treatment of hypertension in adults (2021). Public PDF: who.int (Accessed 2025-08-16).

6. Public Health Agency of Canada (PHAC). High blood pressure—overview & prevention (updated 2025). Public: canada.ca (Accessed 2025-08-16).

ATRIAL FIBRILLATION — FAMILY MEDICINE OFFICE

OVERVIEW & "DON'T MISS"

1. AF is the most common sustained arrhythmia; goals: symptom control (rate/rhythm) + stroke prevention + comorbidity management.
2. Classify: new-onset; paroxysmal (<7 d, self-terminating); persistent (>7 d or cardioversion needed); permanent (accepted).
3. DON'T MISS: hemodynamic instability (hypotension, ischemia, acute HF, syncope), AF with WPW/ pre-excitation (avoid AV-nodal blockers), stroke/TIA symptoms, sepsis/PE/thyrotoxicosis triggers.

HISTORY & EXAM

1. Symptoms: palpitations, dyspnea, fatigue/exercise intolerance, chest discomfort, dizziness/syncope; onset/duration.
2. Triggers/comorbidities: alcohol ('holiday heart'), infection, thyroid disease, anemia, OSA, COPD/ asthma, HTN, DM, HF, CAD, valvular disease;

stimulant/caffeine use.

3. Medications: bronchodilators, decongestants, thyroid, anticoagulants/antiplatelets; bleeding history.

4. Exam: vitals incl. BP and O2; irregularly irregular pulse; signs of HF (JVP, edema, rales); thyroid exam; neuro screen for TIA/stroke.

DIFFERENTIAL DIAGNOSIS (TOP 5)

1. Other supraventricular tachyarrhythmias (atrial flutter, MAT).

2. Sinus tachycardia from infection/anemia/thyrotoxicosis/ PE.

3. PACs with bigeminy perceived as irregular pulse.

4. SVT with variable AV block; AF with pre-excitation (irregular wide-complex).

5. Frequent PVCs/VT in structural heart disease.

INVESTIGATIONS (POC/LABS/IMAGING)

1. 12-lead ECG (confirm AF, rate, QRS, QT, pre-excitation; look for flutter sawtooth). Consider rhythm strip/ambulatory monitor if intermittent.

2. Labs: CBC (anemia), BMP (K/Mg/Cr), TSH, ± troponin if ischemia, LFTs if planning DOAC; A1C/lipids for risk. Pregnancy test if applicable.

3. CXR if HF/respiratory symptoms; transthoracic echo (TTE) to assess structure/function (valve disease, LV function, LA size) — refer if not immediately available.

4. Stroke & bleeding risk: CHA_2DS_2-VASc; HAS-BLED (to identify modifiable risks, not to deny anticoagulation).

MANAGEMENT (NON-PHARM → MEDS → PROCEDURES)

A. NON-PHARMACOLOGIC

1. ABC pathway: A — Avoid stroke (anticoagulate as indicated); B — Better symptom control (rate/rhythm); C — Cardiovascular risk/comorbidity optimization (BP, DM, OSA, weight, exercise, alcohol reduction, smoking cessation).
2. Patient education: pulse checks, anticoagulation adherence, bleeding precautions, when to seek urgent care.

B. MEDICATIONS (EXAMPLES; INDIVIDUALIZE)

1. Stroke prevention (non-valvular AF):
2. Use CHA_2DS_2-VASc (C1, H1, A2 ≥75 =2, D1, S2 stroke/TIA=2, V1, A1 65–74, Sc sex female=1). Anticoagulate: men ≥2, women ≥3; consider men 1/ women 2 after discussion. Female sex alone is not an indication.
3. Prefer DOACs over warfarin unless mechanical valve or moderate-to-severe mitral stenosis (then warfarin; target INR per valve).
4. Typical DOAC dosing (verify local monographs/renal function):

5. – Apixaban 5 mg BID (2.5 mg BID if ≥2 of: age ≥80, weight ≤60 kg, or Cr ≥133 µmol/L/1.5 mg/dL; consider 2.5 mg BID if CrCl 15–29 mL/min).

6. – Rivaroxaban 20 mg daily with food (CrCl 15–50 → 15 mg daily; avoid <15).

7. – Dabigatran 150 mg BID (consider 110 mg BID age ≥80 or ↑bleed risk; avoid CrCl <30).

8. Concomitant antiplatelet generally not needed unless clear indication (recent ACS/stent). Use PPI if GI bleed risk.

9. Rate control:

10. First-line: β-blocker (e.g., metoprolol) OR diltiazem/ verapamil if no HFrEF; goal resting HR often <100– 110 (lenient control).

11. HFrEF (LVEF ≤40%): use β-blocker; avoid diltiazem/ verapamil. Add digoxin if needed (monitor level/renal).

12. Rhythm control (consider early in symptomatic, new-onset, or HF):

13. Antiarrhythmics: no structural heart disease — flecainide/propafenone; with CAD/HF — amiodarone preferred; sotalol requires QT/renal monitoring. Initiation often with cardiology.

14. 'Pill-in-the-pocket' single-dose flecainide/propafenone for selected patients after cardiology-supervised test dose; ensure AV-nodal blocker on board.

15. Cardioversion: if AF >48 h or unknown duration → ≥3 weeks therapeutic anticoagulation or TEE-guided;

continue anticoagulation ≥4 weeks after, and long-term per CHA$_2$DS$_2$-VASc regardless of apparent rhythm outcome.

C. PROCEDURES

1. Office: 12-lead ECG, ambulatory monitoring orders, initiate/adjust rate control and anticoagulation.

2. Refer for: elective cardioversion, ablation for symptomatic AF failure of meds, evaluation of suspected structural heart disease, or consideration of left atrial appendage occlusion (when long-term OAC contraindicated).

DISPOSITION (DISCHARGE/OBSERVE/ TRANSFER) & RETURN PRECAUTIONS

1. Discharge with plan if stable: start/adjust rate control, initiate anticoagulation when indicated, arrange echo and cardiology follow-up; reassess within 1–4 weeks.

2. Same-day/ED: hemodynamic instability, ischemia, decompensated HF, AF with pre-excitation (irregular wide-complex tachycardia), stroke/TIA symptoms, severe dyspnea, syncope.

3. Return urgently for: chest pain, new/worsening dyspnea, syncope, neurological deficit, or bleeding on anticoagulant.

PEARLS & PITFALLS

1. Do not withhold anticoagulation solely for HAS-BLED

≥3 — instead correct modifiable risks (BP, alcohol, NSAIDs, labile INRs).

2. Check renal/hepatic function at baseline and at least annually (more often if CKD/elderly) to ensure correct DOAC dosing.

3. Avoid AV-nodal blockers in AF with WPW/ pre-excitation — seek urgent cardiology.

4. Screen/treat OSA, manage weight, and limit alcohol — these substantially reduce AF recurrence.

5. After cardioversion, continue OAC ≥4 weeks and then by CHA_2DS_2-VASc, not by perceived maintenance of sinus rhythm.

REFERENCES

1. NICE Guideline NG196. Atrial fibrillation: diagnosis and management (open). nice.org.uk

2. Canadian Cardiovascular Society (CCS). Atrial Fibrillation Guidelines (open summaries/updates). ccs.ca

3. Thrombosis Canada. Atrial Fibrillation — Stroke Prevention and DOAC Dosing Guides (open). thrombosiscanada.ca

4. AHA/ACC/HRS. 2019–2023 AF Focused Updates/ Guideline (public executive summaries). heart.org / acc.org

5. ESC. 2020 AF guideline key points and patient materials (open). escardio.org

6. BC Guidelines. Atrial Fibrillation Primary Care Pathway

(public). bcguidelines.gov.bc.ca

7. Choosing Wisely Canada. AF and anticoagulation recommendations (public). choosingwiselycanada.org

COMMON CARDIAC CONDTIONS: HEART FAILURE & CORONARY ARTERY DISEASE

OVERVIEW & "DON'T MISS"

1. HF: clinical syndrome from structural/functional cardiac disorder → dyspnea, edema, fatigue. Types: HFrEF (LVEF ≤40%), HFmrEF (41–49%), HFpEF (≥50%).

2. CAD (chronic coronary disease): atherosclerotic plaque with or without prior ACS/PCI/CABG causing angina, dyspnea, or silent ischemia.

3. DON'T MISS: acute coronary syndrome (ACS/STEMI/ NSTEMI), cardiogenic shock, acute decompensated HF with hypoxia, new rapid AF with instability, hypertensive emergency, aortic dissection, pulmonary embolism.

HISTORY & EXAM

1. HF symptoms: exertional dyspnea, orthopnea/PND, ankle swelling, rapid weight gain, fatigue, cough. CAD/ angina: exertional chest pressure/tightness radiating to arm/jaw; relieved by rest/NTG; note atypical symptoms (dyspnea, epigastric pain).

2. Risk factors: age, HTN, DM, CKD, smoking, dyslipidemia, obesity, OSA, family history premature CAD, chemo (anthracyclines), alcohol/cocaine, thyroid disease.

3. Exam: vitals incl. SpO_2; signs of fluid overload (JVP, rales, S3, edema, hepatomegaly) or hypoperfusion (cool extremities). Cardiac exam, lung crackles/wheeze, murmurs (MR/AS), bruits, peripheral pulses; weight trends.

DIFFERENTIAL DIAGNOSIS (TOP 5)

1. Dyspnea/edema: COPD/asthma, pneumonia, PE, nephrotic/cirrhosis, hypothyroidism/anemia.

2. Chest pain: GERD/esophageal spasm, costochondritis, pericarditis/myocarditis, PE, aortic dissection.

INVESTIGATIONS (POC/LABS/IMAGING)

1. ECG for all suspected HF/CAD; chest X-ray if dyspnea/edema; natriuretic peptides (BNP/NT-proBNP) to support/exclude HF; high-sensitivity troponin if acute chest pain or decompensation.

2. Labs: CBC (anemia), CMP ($Cr/K^+/Na$), A1C, fasting lipid panel, TSH, LFTs, ferritin/TSAT (HF iron deficiency). Consider urinalysis (protein) and Mg.

3. Echocardiogram to confirm LVEF/structure if new/worsening HF; repeat if clinical change. Consider ischemic evaluation (stress test or CT coronary

angiography) in stable chest pain per risk; urgent ED pathway for high-risk.

4. Use validated tools: HEART score (ED), ASCVD risk estimator (prevention), CCS angina classification; NYHA class for HF symptoms.

MANAGEMENT (NON-PHARM → MEDS → PROCEDURES)

A. NON-PHARMACOLOGIC

1. Lifestyle/secondary prevention: smoking cessation; Mediterranean-style diet; sodium awareness (avoid high-salt processed foods; individualized restriction); daily weights (report gain ≥1–2 kg in 2–3 days); fluid restriction only if severe hyponatremia or advanced HF.

2. Exercise: cardiac rehab/structured activity as tolerated for stable HF/CAD; avoid strenuous activity during unstable periods.

3. Vaccines: influenza, COVID-19, pneumococcal; consider RSV vaccine per age/eligibility.

4. Education: nitroglycerin use for angina; when to call EMS; avoid NSAIDs which worsen HF and increase CV risk.

B. MEDICATIONS — HF (INITIATE & UP-TITRATE; CHECK BP/CR/K AT BASELINE AND AFTER CHANGES)

1. HFrEF cornerstone ('quadruple therapy'):

2. ARNI (sacubitril/valsartan) preferred; if not feasible → ACEI (e.g., lisinopril) or ARB (e.g., valsartan).

3. Evidence-based β-blocker: carvedilol, metoprolol succinate, or bisoprolol.

4. Mineralocorticoid receptor antagonist (spironolactone/eplerenone) if eGFR ≥30 and K^+ ≤5.0.

5. SGLT2 inhibitor (dapagliflozin or empagliflozin) for all symptomatic HFrEF regardless of diabetes.

6. Loop diuretics (furosemide/bumetanide) for congestion (adjust to weight/symptoms).

7. Add-ons by phenotype: hydralazine/isosorbide dinitrate for Black patients with HFrEF on optimal therapy or ACEI/ARB intolerance; ivabradine for sinus rhythm HR ≥70 despite β-blocker; digoxin in selected persistent symptoms; IV iron for iron deficiency.

8. HFpEF/HFmrEF: control BP (ACEI/ARB/ARNI), diuretics for congestion, SGLT2 inhibitor for all symptomatic HFpEF; consider MRA in selected; manage AF/ischemia/obesity/OSA.

C. MEDICATIONS — CHRONIC CAD (SECONDARY PREVENTION & ANGINA)

1. Antiplatelet: low-dose aspirin 75–100 mg daily for established CAD unless contraindicated. After PCI/ACS, P2Y12 duration per cardiology; avoid routine dual therapy long-term without indication.

2. Lipid lowering: high-intensity statin (atorvastatin 40–80 mg or rosuvastatin 20–40 mg). If LDL-C remains ≥1.8 mmol/L (70 mg/dL) add ezetimibe; consider PCSK9

inhibitor in very-high risk.

3. BP/RAAS: target <130/80 mmHg for most; ACEI/ARB indicated with HF, DM, CKD, or HTN; consider ARNI if HF coexists.

4. Glycemia (with T2D): SGLT2 inhibitor and/or GLP-1 RA with CV benefit irrespective of baseline A1C; individualize A1C (~7% for many).

5. Antianginals: first-line β-blocker; add long-acting CCB or long-acting nitrate if persistent; consider ranolazine if refractory (QT caution). Short-acting nitroglycerin 0.3–0.4 mg SL PRN chest pain; repeat q5 min up to 3 doses — call EMS after first dose if pain severe/persists >5 min. Avoid with PDE-5 inhibitors.

6. Smoking cessation meds: varenicline/bupropion SR/NRT; refer to quit programs.

D. PROCEDURES/REFERRALS

1. Refer to cardiology for new HFrEF, unclear HF etiology, refractory symptoms, recurrent hospitalizations, or consideration of devices (ICD/CRT) and for ischemia testing/revascularization decisions.

2. Order transthoracic echocardiogram for new HF; stress test/CTCA for stable chest pain per risk. Cardiac rehab referral after MI/revascularization or for stable symptomatic HF.

DISPOSITION (DISCHARGE/OBSERVE/ TRANSFER) & RETURN PRECAUTIONS

1. Immediate ED/transfer: chest pain at rest >20 min or with diaphoresis/ECG changes; positive troponin; acute pulmonary edema (rest dyspnea, SpO_2 <90%); syncope with suspected arrhythmia; new confusion/ hypotension; suspected PE/aortic dissection.

2. Same-week follow-up after med changes or new HF diagnosis; nurse/telehealth check for weight/BP/ symptoms.

3. Return immediately for: weight gain ≥2–3 lb (1–1.5 kg) overnight or ≥5 lb (2–3 kg) in a week, worsening orthopnea/PND, new edema, chest pain, palpitations/ syncope.

PEARLS & PITFALLS

1. Start low, go slow — but aim for guideline-directed targets as tolerated; up-titrate every 2–4 weeks.

2. Recheck K^+/Cr 1–2 weeks after starting/up-titrating RAASi/MRA; watch for hyperkalemia and renal function changes.

3. Avoid NSAIDs (fluid retention, renal injury, ↑ CV risk) and most TZDs in HF; use acetaminophen for pain when possible.

4. Many HF/HFpEF patients benefit from SGLT2 inhibitors even without diabetes.

5. Prescribe a nitroglycerin plan and teach patients when to call EMS; review interactions with PDE-5 inhibitors.

REFERENCES

1. AHA/ACC/HFSA 2022 Guideline for the Management of Heart Failure (open access). ahajournals.org

2. AHA/ACC 2023 Guideline for the Management of Patients With Chronic Coronary Disease (public summaries/open). ahajournals.org

3. AHA/ACC 2021 Guideline for the Evaluation and Diagnosis of Chest Pain (open access). ahajournals. org

4. NICE CKS/Guidelines. Heart failure; Angina; Acute coronary syndromes; Chronic heart disease (public). cks.nice.org.uk / nice.org.uk

5. ESC Guidelines 2021–2023: Heart Failure; Chronic Coronary Syndromes (open PDFs). escardio.org

6. AAFP. Heart Failure with Reduced Ejection Fraction: GDMT Overview; Stable Coronary Artery Disease in Primary Care (open articles). aafp.org

7. CDC. Vaccination guidance and smoking cessation resources for cardiovascular patients (public). cdc.gov

ENDOCRINE & METABOLIC

DO NOT MISS ENDOCRINE DISORDERS — RED FLAGS IN FAMILY OFFICE

OVERVIEW & "DON'T MISS"

1. Life-threatening endocrine emergencies can masquerade as infection or cardiac/neurologic disease — recognize early, stabilize, and transfer.

2. Big 7 to know: (1) Diabetic ketoacidosis (DKA), (2) Hyperosmolar hyperglycemic state (HHS), (3) Adrenal crisis, (4) Thyroid storm, (5) Myxedema coma, (6) Hypercalcemic crisis, (7) Pituitary apoplexy. Also: severe hypoglycemia; severe hyponatremia due to endocrine causes (AI/hypothyroid/SIADH).

3. DON'T MISS clues: polyuria/polydipsia + abdominal pain/vomiting; confusion/coma; fever + tachyarrhythmia with tremor and diarrhea; hypothermia/bradycardia/hypoventilation; severe hypotension with hyperpigmentation; back/ head pain with vision loss; dehydration with stones-bones-groans; seizures from hyponatremia.

HISTORY & EXAM

1. Timeline & precipitant: infection, MI, stroke, recent surgery, pregnancy/post-partum, steroid withdrawal/ non-adherence, iodinated contrast, amiodarone, lithium, antipsychotics, diuretics.

2. Symptoms: polyuria/polydipsia, weight loss; heat/ cold intolerance; GI upset; salt craving; headaches/ visual loss; neck pain; weakness/myalgias; confusion/ seizures.

3. Exam: vitals (fever/hypothermia, tachycardia/ bradycardia, hypotension), volume status, Kussmaul respirations, goiter/ophthalmopathy, hyperpigmentation, abdominal tenderness, neurologic deficits, visual fields, back/spine tenderness.

DIFFERENTIAL DIAGNOSIS (TOP 5)

1. Sepsis/SIRS vs endocrine crisis (check glucose/ TSH-FT4/cortisol).

2. DKA/HHS vs alcoholic/starvation ketoacidosis vs toxic ingestions.

3. Thyroid storm vs sympathomimetic toxidrome/ serotonin syndrome/heat stroke.

4. Myxedema coma vs sedative/opioid toxicity vs sepsis vs hypothermia exposure.

5. Adrenal crisis vs hemorrhagic shock vs anaphylaxis; pituitary apoplexy vs subarachnoid hemorrhage/stroke.

INVESTIGATIONS (POC/LABS/IMAGING)

1. POC glucose for all altered/ill patients; capillary β-hydroxybutyrate if available; ECG (QT, arrhythmia, ischemia).

2. Labs (don't delay stabilization/transfer): BMP (Na/K/Cl/ HCO_3, anion gap), Mg/PO_4, serum osmolality, venous/ arterial blood gas, ketones; CBC, CRP; lactate; TSH/ free T4 (± free T3 if storm); random cortisol (draw before steroids if no delay) ± ACTH; troponin if indicated; pregnancy test.

3. Urinalysis/urine ketones; blood/urine cultures if febrile. Corrected sodium in hyperglycemia = measured Na + 1.6–2.4 mmol/L per 5.6 mmol/L (100 mg/dL) glucose rise.

4. Imaging: CXR if infection; non-contrast head CT then MRI pituitary if apoplexy suspected; neck US not urgent in storm; POCUS IVC if skilled (volume).

MANAGEMENT (NON-PHARM → MEDS → PROCEDURES)

A. NON-PHARMACOLOGIC (INITIAL STABILIZATION FOR ALL)

1. ABCs, high-flow oxygen if hypoxic; two large-bore IVs; cardiac monitor; fingerstick glucose; treat hypoglycemia immediately (see below).

2. Fluids: begin isotonic saline for shock/dehydration unless CHF/ESRD; monitor urine output; place patient

NPO until stabilized.

3. Early EMS/ED transfer after initial steps; do not delay for non-critical tests.

B. MEDICATIONS (CONDITION-SPECIFIC FIRST STEPS — OFFICE SCOPE; VERIFY LOCAL PROTOCOLS)

1. Severe hypoglycemia (any cause): if awake — 15–20 g fast carbs; recheck in 15 min. If altered — glucagon 1 mg IM/IN; if IV access — D50W 25 g IV (or D10W infusion). Identify cause; consider octreotide for sulfonylurea-induced (ED).

2. DKA/HHS: start 0.9% saline 1–1.5 L in first hour (adjust for age/CHF). Check K^+ before insulin. If K^+ <3.3 → replete K^+ first. Arrange ED for insulin infusion (0.1 U/kg/h), K^+ replacement, add dextrose when glucose <11–14 mmol/L (200–250 mg/dL).

3. Adrenal crisis: do NOT delay — hydrocortisone 100 mg IV/IM stat then 50 mg IV q6h (or 200 mg/24 h infusion); 1–3 L isotonic saline (add dextrose if hypoglycemic). Draw cortisol first only if it does not delay steroid. Treat precipitant.

4. Thyroid storm: β-block (propranolol 60–80 mg PO q4–6h or esmolol IV), thionamide (PTU 200–250 mg PO q4h OR methimazole 20 mg PO q4–6h), then iodine 1 h later (SSKI 5 drops q6h or Lugol's). Hydrocortisone 100 mg IV q8h; acetaminophen/cooling (avoid salicylates). ED/ICU.

5. Myxedema coma: hydrocortisone 100 mg IV q8h; IV

levothyroxine 200–400 mcg loading then 50–100 mcg daily (± low-dose liothyronine per specialist). Passive rewarming; cautious fluids; correct hyponatremia/hypoglycemia. ED/ICU.

6. Hypercalcemic crisis (Ca □3.5 mmol/L / 14 mg/dL or symptomatic): aggressive IV isotonic saline; calcitonin 4 IU/kg SC/IM q12h; IV bisphosphonate (zoledronic acid 4 mg or pamidronate) via ED; stop thiazides/lithium; consider steroids if calcitriol-mediated.

7. Pituitary apoplexy: hydrocortisone 100 mg IV stat; head CT (rule hemorrhage) then urgent MRI; neurosurg/ophthalmology; manage BP/electrolytes. Avoid delaying steroids.

C. PROCEDURES

1. Give IM hydrocortisone 100 mg immediately for suspected adrenal crisis if IV access delayed.

2. Administer glucagon IM/IN for severe hypoglycemia if no IV access; prepare D50W if IV established.

3. Start aggressive oral/IV fluids while arranging transfer (unless CHF/ESRD—adjust and monitor).

DISPOSITION (DISCHARGE/OBSERVE/ TRANSFER) & RETURN PRECAUTIONS

1. Immediate ED/ICU transfer for all suspected endocrine emergencies above.

2. Outpatient follow-up only after ED evaluation for: mild, resolved hypoglycemia with clear cause and

education; otherwise admit/observe.

3. Return immediately for: persistent vomiting, confusion, chest pain, syncope, seizures, dyspnea, fever, or inability to keep fluids/meds down.

PEARLS & PITFALLS

1. Treat first, confirm later: steroids for adrenal crisis; glucose for hypoglycemia; fluids for DKA/HHS/ hypercalcemia — do not wait for full labs.

2. Correct sodium for hyperglycemia; avoid rapid Na^+ correction in hyponatremia (consult ED for 3% saline bolus if seizures/coma).

3. In thyroid storm: thionamide $\rightarrow$ iodine sequence (iodine 1 h AFTER thionamide) to block hormone release; avoid aspirin (displaces T4/T3).

4. In myxedema coma: passive, not active, rewarming; give steroids before thyroid hormone if AI not excluded.

5. Known Addison's: ensure emergency IM hydrocortisone kit and sick-day rules (double/triple dose during illness).

REFERENCES

1. American Diabetes Association (ADA). Standards of Medical Care in Diabetes — Hyperglycemic Crises in Adults (open access). diabetesjournals.org

2. Joint British Diabetes Societies (JBDS). Management of Diabetic Ketoacidosis and HHS guidelines (open

PDFs). abcd.care/jbds

3. Endocrine Society Clinical Practice Guideline (2016). Diagnosis and Treatment of Primary Adrenal Insufficiency — open summary. endocrine.org

4. Society for Endocrinology (UK). Emergency guidance: Adrenal crisis; Pituitary apoplexy (open PDFs). endocrinology.org

5. American Thyroid Association (ATA). Hyperthyroidism and Other Causes of Thyrotoxicosis (2016) — public resources; and patient/clinician summaries on thyroid storm & myxedema coma. thyroid.org

6. AAFP. Myxedema Coma; Thyroid Storm; Hypercalcemia of Malignancy; Adrenal Insufficiency; Hypoglycemia in Adults (open articles). aafp.org

7. NICE CKS. Hyponatraemia; Hypercalcaemia; Adrenal insufficiency; Diabetic ketoacidosis (public). cks.nice. org.uk

DYSLIPIDEMIA

OVERVIEW & "DON'T MISS"

1. Goal: reduce ASCVD events via lifestyle and lipid-lowering therapy. Focus on risk-based statin therapy, and consider nonstatins when LDL-C remains above threshold despite maximally tolerated statin.

2. Risk categories (adults 40–75 y): use pooled cohort equations (PCE) to estimate 10-yr ASCVD risk: <5% low; 5–7.4% borderline; 7.5–19.9% intermediate; ≥20% high.

3. Automatic indications: clinical ASCVD (secondary prevention), LDL-C ≥190 mg/dL (≥4.9 mmol/L), and diabetes age 40–75 (most need ≥moderate intensity).

4. DON'T MISS: familial hypercholesterolemia (FH) (LDL-C ≥190 mg/dL esp. young, tendon xanthomas, strong FHx), severe hypertriglyceridemia (≥500 mg/dL; ≥11.3 mmol/L) with pancreatitis risk, secondary causes (hypothyroidism, nephrotic syndrome, cholestasis, CKD, pregnancy, excess alcohol, meds like isotretinoin/antipsychotics).

HISTORY & EXAM

1. ASCVD risk: prior MI/stroke/PAD; angina; family history premature ASCVD (men <55, women <65); smoking; HTN; diabetes; CKD; inflammatory diseases (psoriasis, RA); premature menopause/preeclampsia.

2. Diet (saturated/trans fat, refined carbs), alcohol, activity/sedentary time; weight history; adherence and prior statin tolerance (myalgias).

3. Exam: BMI/waist; BP; xanthomas/xanthelasma/corneal arcus (early); pulses/bruits; signs of hypothyroidism or liver disease.

DIFFERENTIAL DIAGNOSIS (TOP 5)

1. Primary hypercholesterolemia (including FH).

2. Combined hyperlipidemia (mixed).

3. Secondary dyslipidemia (hypothyroid, nephrotic, cholestasis, CKD, meds, alcohol).

4. Hypertriglyceridemia (metabolic syndrome, diabetes, alcohol, genetic).

5. Physiologic/pregnancy-related lipid changes.

INVESTIGATIONS (POC/LABS/IMAGING)

1. Lipid panel (non-fasting acceptable for routine; fasting if TG ≥400 mg/dL or to diagnose severe HTG). Measure baseline and 4–12 weeks after therapy changes, then q3–12 months.

2. Secondary causes: TSH, A1C/fasting glucose, CMP (ALT/AST, creatinine), urine ACR if CKD suspected;

consider nephrotic work-up if edema/proteinuria.

3. Risk-enhancing factors (support statin at borderline/ intermediate risk): family history premature ASCVD, LDL-C 160–189 mg/dL, metabolic syndrome, CKD, inflammatory diseases, South Asian ancestry, triglycerides ≥175 mg/dL, elevated Lp(a) (≥50 mg/dL or ≥125 nmol/L), ApoB ≥130 mg/dL, hs-CRP ≥2 mg/L.

4. If risk decision uncertain: Coronary artery calcium (CAC) scoring — CAC=0 may allow deferral in some (except smokers, diabetes, strong FHx); CAC ≥100 or ≥75th percentile strongly favors statin.

MANAGEMENT (NON-PHARM → MEDS → PROCEDURES)

A. NON-PHARMACOLOGIC

1. Diet: Mediterranean/DASH emphasis; replace saturated with mono/poly-unsaturated fats; increase soluble fiber (oats, legumes), nuts, plant sterols; reduce refined carbs/sugary drinks; limit alcohol (especially if TG high).

2. Weight: aim ≥5–10% loss if overweight/obesity; address sleep/OSA; smoking cessation; ≥150 min/wk moderate-vigorous aerobic + 2–3 resistance sessions.

3. Manage comorbidities: optimize diabetes/BP; treat hypothyroidism; review meds that raise lipids.

B. MEDICATIONS — STATINS (FIRST-LINE)

1. Intensity & typical doses:

2. HIGH: atorvastatin 40–80 mg; rosuvastatin 20–40 mg ($\downarrow$ LDL-C ≥50%).

3. MODERATE: atorvastatin 10–20 mg; rosuvastatin 5–10 mg; simvastatin 20–40 mg; pravastatin 40–80 mg; lovastatin 40 mg; fluvastatin XL 80 mg; pitavastatin 2–4 mg ($\downarrow$ 30–49%).

4. LOW: simvastatin 10 mg; pravastatin 10–20 mg; lovastatin 20 mg; fluvastatin 20–40 mg; pitavastatin 1 mg ($\downarrow$ <30%).

5. Monitoring: check fasting/nonfasting lipid panel 4–12 wks after start/titration; ALT at baseline and if symptoms; CK only if muscle symptoms. Counsel on myalgias; watch interactions (macrolides, azoles, cyclosporine, grapefruits for some).

6. Pregnancy/breastfeeding: generally avoid statins; use bile-acid sequestrants if needed (specialist).

C. WHEN TO ADD NONSTATINS (EXAMPLES; VERIFY COVERAGE/COST)

1. SECONDARY PREVENTION (clinical ASCVD): high-intensity statin → if LDL-C ≥70 mg/dL (1.8 mmol/L) or non-HDL ≥100 mg/dL despite max tolerated statin: add ezetimibe 10 mg daily. If still above threshold (esp. very-high risk): add PCSK9 inhibitor (alirocumab/evolocumab).

2. PRIMARY PREVENTION — LDL-C ≥190 mg/dL: high-intensity statin → if LDL-C remains ≥100 mg/dL (2.6 mmol/L), add ezetimibe; consider PCSK9 inhibitor in FH if persistent elevation.

3. PRIMARY PREVENTION — Diabetes 40–75 y: at least moderate-intensity; if multiple risk factors or age 50–75, consider high-intensity; add ezetimibe if needed for goals.

4. PRIMARY PREVENTION — Borderline/intermediate risk with high risk-enhancers or CAC ≥100: consider starting or intensifying statin; ezetimibe add-on if LDL-C above shared goal.

5. Additional agents:

6. Bempedoic acid 180 mg daily (oral) for statin-intolerant or add-on (↓ LDL ~15–25%).

7. Inclisiran 284 mg SC day 0, 3 months, then q6 months (↓ LDL ~50% when added to statin).

8. PCSK9 mAbs (alirocumab 75–150 mg q2–4w; evolocumab 140 mg q2w or 420 mg monthly).

D. TRIGLYCERIDES

1. TG 150–499 mg/dL (1.7–5.6 mmol/L): lifestyle first (weight loss, less refined carbs/alcohol); optimize statin if ASCVD risk. Consider icosapent ethyl 2 g BID for patients with established ASCVD or diabetes + risk factors on statin with TG 135–499 mg/dL (reduces CV events).

2. TG ≥500 mg/dL (≥5.6 mmol/L): pancreatitis risk — very low-fat diet, eliminate alcohol/refined carbs; initiate fibrate (fenofibrate preferred with statin) and/or high-dose omega-3; control diabetes and hypothyroidism; consider inpatient if TG ≥1000 with symptoms.

3. Avoid gemfibrozil with statins when possible (rhabdomyolysis risk).

DISPOSITION (DISCHARGE/OBSERVE/ TRANSFER) & RETURN PRECAUTIONS

1. Emergency: abdominal pain/vomiting with very high TG (suspect pancreatitis) — send to ED.

2. Urgent specialty referral: suspected FH, statin intolerance with recurrent myopathy after trials, LDL-C not at threshold despite 2+ agents, TG ≥1000 mg/dL, pregnancy with severe dyslipidemia, complex polypharmacy interactions.

3. Follow-up: recheck lipids 4–12 wks after changes, then q3–12 months; reinforce adherence and lifestyle; monitor for adverse effects (myopathy, new diabetes risk minimal vs benefits).

PEARLS & PITFALLS

1. Use shared decision-making with risk discussion, especially for borderline/intermediate risk and for adding nonstatins.

2. Consider ApoB or non-HDL-C as alternative targets in hypertriglyceridemia or mixed dyslipidemia.

3. Order Lp(a) once in a lifetime (family history or premature ASCVD) to refine risk — no specific therapy yet, but guides intensity.

4. CAC scoring helps avoid both undertreatment and overtreatment when PCE risk is uncertain.

5. Address adherence first when LDL-C not at goal — missed doses are common.

REFERENCES

1. AHA/ACC 2018 Guideline on the Management of Blood Cholesterol (open access). ahajournals.org

2. ACC 2022 Expert Consensus Decision Pathway on the Role of Nonstatin Therapies for LDL-C Lowering (open access). jacc.org

3. USPSTF 2022 Recommendation: Statin Use for the Primary Prevention of Cardiovascular Disease in Adults (public). uspreventiveservicestaskforce.org

4. NICE CKS. Lipid modification — cardiovascular risk assessment and management (public). cks.nice.org.uk

5. ESC/EAS 2019 Guidelines for the management of dyslipidaemias (open PDF). escardio.org

6. AAFP. Cholesterol Management: ACC/AHA Updates; Hypertriglyceridemia: Management of Elevated Triglycerides (open articles). aafp.org

7. FDA. Statins: information on use in pregnancy and safety communications (public). fda.gov

TYPE 2 DIABETES — FAMILY MEDICINE OFFICE

OVERVIEW & "DON'T MISS"

1. Chronic, progressive metabolic disease with high cardiometabolic risk; aim for glycemic control + weight management + cardio-renal protection.

2. Targets (individualize): A1C ~7% for most (less stringent in frailty/hypoglycemia risk), BP <130/80 mmHg for many, LDL-C per ASCVD risk (high-intensity statin in most ≥40 y with diabetes).

3. DON'T MISS: diabetic ketoacidosis (may be euglycemic with SGLT2i), hyperosmolar hyperglycemic state (HHS), severe hypoglycemia, ACS/stroke, foot infection/critical limb ischemia, vision loss, rapidly progressive kidney disease, new insulin-deficient diabetes (type 1/LADA).

HISTORY & EXAM

1. Symptoms: polyuria/polydipsia, weight change, fatigue, blurred vision, infections/slow healing, neuropathic pain, claudication, angina/SOB, nocturia.

2. Lifestyle & context: diet pattern, physical activity, sleep/OSA, alcohol/tobacco, psychosocial barriers, health literacy, access/costs.

3. Complications review: hypoglycemia awareness, CV history (ASCVD/HF), CKD, eye disease, neuropathy, sexual/urogenital health, foot ulcers.

4. Meds: steroids/atypical antipsychotics; adherence; adverse effects.

5. Exam: BMI/waist, BP (sitting/standing), fundi (if trained), thyroid/skin (acanthosis), feet (monofilament/vibration, pulses, skin), injection sites if using insulin/GLP-1.

DIFFERENTIAL DIAGNOSIS (TOP 5)

1. Type 1 diabetes or LADA (autoimmune; ketones, weight loss, low/normal BMI).

2. Pancreatogenic (type 3c) from pancreatitis/pancreatectomy.

3. Medication-induced (glucocorticoids, HAART, atypical antipsychotics).

4. Endocrine: Cushing syndrome, acromegaly, pheochromocytoma, hyperthyroidism.

5. Monogenic diabetes (MODY) in young, non-obese with strong FHx.

INVESTIGATIONS (POC/LABS/IMAGING)

1. Diagnosis (repeat to confirm unless unequivocal hyperglycemia): A1C ≥6.5%; OR FPG ≥126 mg/

dL (7.0 mmol/L); OR 2-h OGTT ≥200 mg/dL (11.1 mmol/L); OR random glucose ≥200 mg/dL with classic symptoms.

2. Baseline/ongoing labs: A1C q3 months if not at goal (q6 months when stable); fasting lipids; serum creatinine/eGFR; urine albumin-to-creatinine ratio (UACR) yearly; LFTs; B12 periodically if on metformin; TSH if symptoms; consider ALT/AST for MASLD risk.

3. Screen complications: dilated retinal exam at diagnosis then q1–2 y; comprehensive foot exam yearly (or each visit if high risk); neuropathy screen (monofilament/ vibration); BP every visit; ECG if CV symptoms.

4. Vaccines: influenza, COVID-19, pneumococcal (PCV20 or PCV15→PPSV23 per program), hepatitis B; consider zoster per age.

5. Technology: consider intermittent or real-time CGM to reduce hypoglycemia and support titration, especially on insulin or sulfonylureas.

MANAGEMENT (NON-PHARM → MEDS → PROCEDURES)

A. NON-PHARMACOLOGIC (FOR ALL)

1. Diabetes self-management education/support (DSMES).

2. Nutrition: individualized eating pattern (Mediterranean/ DASH/low-carb/plate method); reduce refined carbs/ sugary drinks; adequate protein; consider dietitian

referral.

3. Weight: aim ≥5–10% loss (≥15% if obesity) via nutrition + activity ± anti-obesity meds or bariatric referral as appropriate.

4. Physical activity: ≥150 min/wk moderate-vigorous aerobic + 2–3 sessions/wk resistance + ↓ sedentary time; assess fall/CV risk before vigorous programs.

5. Foot care daily; smoking cessation; moderate alcohol; sleep optimization; mental health support.

B. GLUCOSE-LOWERING MEDICATIONS (ADULT T2D; INDIVIDUALIZE BY COMORBIDITIES, A1C, COST, PREFERENCES)

1. First-line: Metformin unless contraindicated (eGFR <30). Titrate: 500 mg daily with food → ↑ every 1–2 wks to 1000 mg BID (or XR 2,000 mg daily) as tolerated; GI effects common; monitor B12 long-term.

2. Cardio-renal protection regardless of baseline A1C (if eligible):

3. SGLT2 inhibitor (empagliflozin, dapagliflozin, canagliflozin) for HF (any EF) and CKD with albuminuria; benefits on hospitalization for HF and kidney outcomes. Check eGFR thresholds and hold during acute illness/surgery (DKA risk).

4. GLP-1 receptor agonist (semaglutide, dulaglutide) or dual GIP/GLP-1 agonist (tirzepatide) for ASCVD risk reduction and weight loss; GI effects; avoid with personal/family MTC/MEN2.

5. A1C ≥9% or not at goal after ~3 months: use

dual therapy (metformin + agent above based on comorbidities).

6. If A1C ≥10%, symptomatic hyperglycemia (polyuria/polydipsia/weight loss), or catabolic features → start insulin (± GLP-1 RA) promptly.

7. Other options (consider cost/hypoglycemia/weight): DPP-4 inhibitors (weight-neutral, modest); sulfonylureas (effective, low cost; risk hypoglycemia/weight gain); thiazolidinediones (edema, HF risk, fractures).

8. Basal insulin initiation: start 10 units daily or 0.1–0.2 u/kg; titrate +2 u every 3 days to FBG 80–130 mg/dL (4.4–7.2 mmol/L); address hypoglycemia. Consider adding GLP-1 RA before prandial insulin if post-prandial excursions predominate.

C. CARDIOVASCULAR RISK & CKD MANAGEMENT

1. BP: ACEI/ARB first-line if albuminuria (UACR ≥30 mg/g); add thiazide-like diuretic (chlorthalidone/indapamide) or dihydropyridine CCB as needed.

2. Lipids: high-intensity statin for most adults 40–75 y; add ezetimibe or PCSK9 inhibitor if very high risk and LDL-C above target.

3. Antiplatelet: low-dose aspirin for secondary prevention; consider primary prevention only if high ASCVD risk and low bleeding risk.

4. CKD: SGLT2 inhibitor for UACR ≥200 mg/g (and often even with lower albuminuria if eGFR allows); consider

finerenone (ns-MRA) in persistent albuminuria despite ACEI/ARB (monitor K$^+$).

DISPOSITION (DISCHARGE/OBSERVE/ TRANSFER) & RETURN PRECAUTIONS

1. Same-week ED/urgent care: suspected DKA/HHS (polyuria/polydipsia with vomiting/dehydration, abdominal pain, Kussmaul breathing, confusion), chest pain/neurologic deficits, sepsis/foot infection with systemic signs.

2. Urgent referrals (days–weeks): rapidly rising creatinine or UACR, proliferative retinopathy or acute vision change, recurrent severe hypoglycemia, refractory A1C despite maximal therapy, suspected T1D/LADA, pregnancy planning.

3. Return immediately for: recurrent lows (<70 mg/dL / 3.9 mmol/L), persistent fasting >250 mg/dL (13.9 mmol/L), vomiting/dehydration while on SGLT2i or insulin, foot ulcer/redness/swelling.

PEARLS & PITFALLS

1. Match drug to disease: SGLT2i for HF/CKD; GLP-1 RA/dual incretin for ASCVD/weight; avoid sulfonylureas if hypoglycemia risk.

2. A1C can mislead in anemia/hemoglobinopathies — use SMBG/CGM and fructosamine when needed; CGM time-in-range goal ≥70% (70–180 mg/dL).

3. Sick-day rules: hold metformin with dehydration/

hypoxia/contrast risk; pause SGLT2i during acute illness/surgery; never stop basal insulin entirely.

4. Check feet at every visit; empower self-inspection and footwear advice.

5. Screen and treat depression, OSA, and NAFLD — they worsen glycemic control and CV risk.

REFERENCES

1. American Diabetes Association. Standards of Care in Diabetes — 2024/2025 (open access). diabetesjournals.org/care

2. NICE Guideline NG28. Type 2 diabetes in adults: management (public). nice.org.uk

3. Diabetes Canada Clinical Practice Guidelines (open access). diabetes.ca

4. KDIGO 2022 Diabetes in CKD Guideline (open PDF). kdigo.org

5. AHA/ACC Prevention & Hypertension guidelines relevant to diabetes care (public summaries). ahajournals.org

6. AAFP. Type 2 Diabetes: Outpatient Insulin Management; Cardiovascular Risk Reduction in T2D; GLP-1/SGLT2 Overviews (open articles). aafp.org

7. CDC. Adult Immunization Schedule (public). cdc.gov

INSULIN MANAGEMENT IN TYPE 2 DIABETES

OVERVIEW & "DON'T MISS"

1. When: consider insulin at diagnosis if A1C ≥10% (86 mmol/mol), symptomatic hyperglycemia (polyuria/polydipsia/weight loss), ketonuria, or catabolic features; or when oral/GLP-1/SGLT2 therapies fail to reach individualized targets.

2. Goals (typical): A1C ~7% for most; fasting/pre-meal 4.4–7.2 mmol/L (80–130 mg/dL); 2-h post-meal <10.0 mmol/L (<180 mg/dL). Individualize by age/comorbidity/hypoglycemia risk.

3. DON'T MISS: DKA/HHS, frequent/severe hypoglycemia or hypoglycemia unawareness, insulin pump failure (if using), infection precipitating uncontrolled hyperglycemia, steroid-induced hyperglycemia needing temporary insulin.

HISTORY & EXAM

1. Assess: symptoms (polyuria, nocturia, thirst, weight change), hypoglycemia episodes, food pattern/shift

work, visual impairment/dexterity, cognition/support, comorbidities (CKD/CVD/HF), steroid use, pregnancy plans.

2. Review meds: continue metformin if tolerated; consider continuing SGLT2/GLP-1 RA for CV/renal benefit even with insulin; stop or reduce sulfonylurea/meglitinide when starting prandial insulin to lower hypo risk.

3. Baseline: vitals, weight/BMI, injection sites/skin exam; SMBG or CGM access and ability; vaccination status (influenza, pneumococcal, hepatitis B).

DIFFERENTIAL DIAGNOSIS (TOP 5)

1. Type 1 diabetes or LADA (lean, rapid progression, ketosis) requiring full insulin regimen.

2. Medication-induced hyperglycemia (glucocorticoids, antipsychotics).

3. Hyperthyroidism, Cushing syndrome, acromegaly worsening control.

4. Nonadherence/barriers (cost, technique, depression).

5. Infection causing transient decompensation.

INVESTIGATIONS (POC/LABS/IMAGING)

1. POC glucose and ketones if symptomatic. A1C every 3 months until at goal. BMP (eGFR/K^+), LFTs; lipids annually; urine ACR; TSH if indicated.

2. Consider autoantibodies (GAD65/IA-2/ZnT8) and C-peptide if suspected LADA/Type 1.

3. If using GLP-1/SGLT2 with insulin, monitor renal

function and volume status; educate on sick-day rules.

MANAGEMENT (NON-PHARM → MEDS → PROCEDURES)

A. NON-PHARMACOLOGIC

1. Diabetes self-management education (DSME): injection technique, rotation, storage, disposal; SMBG/ CGM use; hypoglycemia recognition/treatment ('15-15 rule').

2. Nutrition & activity: consistent carbohydrate pattern; medical nutrition therapy; physical activity 150 min/wk as tolerated; weight-focused care (prefer GLP-1 RA/ SGLT2 continuation for weight/CV benefit).

3. Sick-day rules: never stop basal insulin; check glucose q3–4 h (more if unwell); check ketones if glucose persistently >13.9 mmol/L (>250 mg/dL) or sick; hydrate; hold SADMANS as appropriate; seek care for vomiting, ketones, or persistent hyperglycemia.

B. MEDICATIONS — INSULIN ALGORITHMS (EXAMPLES; INDIVIDUALIZE)

1. Start BASAL insulin:

2. Start 10 units once daily OR 0.1–0.2 units/kg/day (NPH at HS or long-acting analog once daily).

3. Titrate: increase by 2 units every 3 days (or 1 unit/day) to fasting 4.4–7.2 mmol/L (80–130 mg/dL); if fasting <3.9 (70) or symptomatic hypo → reduce 10–20%.

4. If basal dose >0.5 units/kg/day and A1C remains above goal → consider post-prandial coverage (GLP-1 RA preferred before bolus insulin for many) or move to basal-bolus/premix.

5. Add PRANDIAL insulin ('basal-plus' then intensify):

6. Start with largest meal: 4 units OR 0.1 units/kg OR 10% of basal dose before meal.

7. Titrate by 1–2 units (or 10–15%) twice weekly to 2-h post-meal <10 mmol/L (<180 mg/dL) without hypo. Add to second/third meals as needed.

8. Full BASAL-BOLUS:

9. Total daily dose (TDD) 0.3–0.5 units/kg/day (lower if elderly/CKD). Split ~50% basal and 50% prandial divided across meals. Adjust using fasting and pre-/post-meal SMBG or CGM.

10. PREMIXED insulin (e.g., 70/30 or 75/25) twice daily if simpler regimen desired:

11. Start 0.3–0.5 units/kg/day → give 2/3 before breakfast and 1/3 before supper; titrate to fasting and pre-supper targets. Less flexible; risk of hypoglycemia if meals skipped.

12. Concentrated basals (e.g., glargine U-300, degludec U-200):

13. Useful for large doses or nocturnal hypoglycemia; dose in units (pen delivers actual units). Expect slower titration and flatter profile.

14. Corrections/ISF (insulin sensitivity factor) for advanced users/CGM:

15. Simple clinic correction scale: add 1–2 units rapid-acting if pre-meal glucose 10–14 mmol/L (180–250), add 2–4 units if 14–17 mmol/L (250–300), and seek advice if higher or ketones present. Individualize based on hypoglycemia history.

16. Concomitant agents with insulin:

17. Continue metformin unless contraindicated. Continue SGLT2 (watch euglycemic DKA risk; hold for surgery/acute illness). GLP-1 RA before or with prandial insulin often improves weight/hypoglycemia profile. Stop or reduce sulfonylurea/meglitinide when adding bolus insulin.

18. Hypoglycemia management & prevention:

19. Treat <3.9 mmol/L (<70 mg/dL) with 15–20 g fast carbs; recheck in 15 min; repeat until >4.0 (72). Prescribe glucagon (nasal/IM) for severe episodes; review pattern/insulin doses, meals, activity, alcohol.

20. Special situations:

21. CKD (eGFR <30): insulin requirements often ↓ — consider 25–50% lower starting doses; prefer long-acting analogs to reduce hypo; closer monitoring.

22. Steroid-induced hyperglycemia: add/adjust NPH in morning (matches prednisone peak) or increase basal/bolus per glucose profile.

23. Peri-procedure/fasting: give 50–80% of usual basal morning of procedure; hold prandial; target 6–10 mmol/L (108–180 mg/dL).

24. Older/frail: higher targets (e.g., fasting 6–9 mmol/L);

prioritize avoiding hypoglycemia; simplify regimen (basal only ± correction).

C. PROCEDURES

1. Teach and document injection technique (pinch, angle, 4–6 mm needles), site rotation (abdomen/thigh/arm), and pen priming; check storage (refrigerate unopened; in-use at room temp per product).

2. Set a written titration plan (patient-driven where possible) and SMBG/CGM schedule; provide hypoglycemia action plan and glucagon kit prescription.

DISPOSITION (DISCHARGE/OBSERVE/ TRANSFER) & RETURN PRECAUTIONS

1. Discharge with: written titration algorithm, SMBG/CGM instructions, follow-up in 1–2 weeks for new starts/ intensifications, and foot/eye screening schedule.

2. Urgent same-day/ED: vomiting with hyperglycemia/ ketones, altered mental status, suspected DKA/ HHS, recurrent severe hypoglycemia, or inability to self-manage safely at home.

PEARLS & PITFALLS

1. If fasting is at target but A1C remains high, problem is post-prandial — add GLP-1 RA or prandial insulin rather than further raising basal ('over-basalization').

2. Match the regimen to the patient: meal regularity

$\rightarrow$ premix may work; variable meals $\rightarrow$ basal-plus is safer; high hypo risk $\rightarrow$ prefer analogs and conservative targets.

3. Stop or reduce sulfonylureas when adding prandial insulin to avoid hypoglycemia.

4. Use CGM or structured SMBG to guide changes; small frequent adjustments work better than rare large ones.

5. Always educate on sick-day rules and never stopping basal insulin.

REFERENCES

1. American Diabetes Association (ADA). Standards of Medical Care in Diabetes — Glycemic Targets and Pharmacologic Approaches (open access). diabetesjournals.org

2. NICE Guideline NG28. Type 2 diabetes in adults: management (public). nice.org.uk

3. Diabetes Canada. Pharmacologic Glycemic Management of Type 2 Diabetes in Adults (open access clinician tools). diabetes.ca

4. AAFP. Outpatient Insulin Management in Type 2 Diabetes; Insulin Therapy for Type 2 Diabetes Mellitus (open articles). aafp.org

5. TREND-UK. Insulin safety guidance and patient education resources (open). trend-uk.org

6. Endocrine Society patient/clinician resources on insulin and hypoglycaemia (public). endocrine.org

COMMON ENDOCRINE DISORDERS IN FAMILY PRACTICE

OVERVIEW & "DON'T MISS"

1. Endocrine disorders often present subtly (weight change, fatigue, resistant hypertension, menstrual/ sexual dysfunction). Use targeted screens for high-yield conditions.

2. Key groups covered here: Primary Aldosteronism (PA), Cushing Syndrome, Pheochromocytoma/ Paraganglioma (PPGL), Primary Hyperparathyroidism (PHPT), Primary Adrenal Insufficiency (AI), Hyperprolactinemia, and Acromegaly.

3. DON'T MISS: adrenal crisis (shock/hypoglycemia), pheochromocytoma crisis (hypertensive emergency), severe hypercalcemia, pituitary apoplexy, and steroid withdrawal.

HISTORY & EXAM

1. PA: resistant HTN (≥3 meds), hypokalemia or diuretic-induced, early-onset HTN, adrenal incidentaloma, sleep apnea, family hx early stroke.

2. Cushing: proximal muscle weakness, easy bruising, wide violaceous striae, facial plethora, dorsocervical fat, weight gain, diabetes/HTN, osteopenia, mood change.

3. PPGL: paroxysmal headaches, palpitations, diaphoresis, pallor; labile HTN; spells with panic-like symptoms; family hx MEN2/SDHx.

4. PHPT: stones, bone pain/fractures, abdominal pain/ constipation, depression/cognitive change; thiazide/ lithium use.

5. AI (Addison): fatigue, weight loss, hyperpigmentation, orthostasis, salt craving, abdominal pain; precipitated by illness/steroid cessation.

6. Hyperprolactinemia: galactorrhea, amenorrhea/ oligomenorrhea, infertility, decreased libido, headaches/visual field defects.

7. Acromegaly: change in ring/shoe size, coarse features, jaw malocclusion, snoring/OSA, carpal tunnel, DM/ HTN, cardiomyopathy.

DIFFERENTIAL DIAGNOSIS (TOP 5)

1. Essential HTN vs. secondary HTN due to PA/PPGL/ CKD/OSA.

2. Pseudo-Cushing states (alcoholism, depression, severe obesity, chronic stress) and exogenous glucocorticoid use.

3. Medication effects: OCPs/estrogens ($\uparrow$CBG), antipsychotics/risperidone/metoclopramide

(↑prolactin), thiazides/lithium (↑Ca), β-blockers/central α-2 (↓renin).

4. Primary hypercalcemia (PHPT) vs malignancy-related hypercalcemia (PTHrP, bone mets, myeloma).

5. Hypogonadism/thyroid disease mimicking hyperprolactinemia or acromegaly symptoms.

INVESTIGATIONS (POC/LABS/IMAGING)

1. Primary Aldosteronism (screen): morning seated aldosterone-renin ratio (ARR). Correct hypokalemia first; liberalize Na for a few days. Hold MRAs (spironolactone/eplerenone) 4–6 wks if feasible; minimize interfering drugs (β-blockers ↓renin; diuretics/ACEi/ARB affect results). Positive screen → confirmatory test (saline/oral salt load) and adrenal imaging ± adrenal vein sampling (AVS).

2. Cushing (screen — choose ONE): 1-mg overnight dex suppression (AM cortisol >1.8 μg/dL [50 nmol/L] positive), OR late-night salivary cortisol (×2), OR 24-h urinary free cortisol (×2). Avoid random cortisol. If positive → ACTH level + further work-up/referral.

3. PPGL: plasma free metanephrines (supine, rested) or 24-h urinary fractionated metanephrines; avoid caffeine/nicotine and certain meds before test; if positive → imaging (MRI abdomen/pelvis or CT).

4. PHPT: elevated or inappropriately normal PTH with high total/ionized calcium; check albumin, eGFR, 25-OH vitamin D, phosphate. Distinguish from FHH using 24-h urine calcium/Cr clearance ratio (FHH low).

5. Primary Adrenal Insufficiency: 8–9 AM serum cortisol + ACTH. If indeterminate, 250-μg cosyntropin test (AI if 30–60-min cortisol fails to rise adequately). Electrolytes: hyponatremia/hyperkalemia; consider 21-hydroxylase antibodies.

6. Hyperprolactinemia: serum prolactin (repeat if mild ↑). Exclude pregnancy, hypothyroidism (TSH), renal failure, meds. If high or symptomatic → pituitary MRI. Beware 'hook effect' in macroprolactinoma (ask lab to dilute).

7. Acromegaly: elevated IGF-1 for age/sex; confirm with failure of GH suppression during 75-g OGTT; pituitary MRI after biochemical diagnosis.

MANAGEMENT (NON-PHARM → MEDS → PROCEDURES)

A. NON-PHARMACOLOGIC

1. Address cardiometabolic risk: BP, lipids, weight, exercise, smoking, sleep apnea. Vaccinate (influenza, pneumococcal, shingles where appropriate).

2. Medication review and deprescribing contributors (e.g., thiazides/lithium in hypercalcemia; antipsychotics/metoclopramide in hyperprolactinemia; estrogen effect on cortisol tests).

B. MEDICATIONS (EXAMPLES; FIRST-LINE/ BRIDGE; SPECIALIST-DIRECTED FOR MANY)

1. Primary Aldosteronism: unilateral adenoma

→ adrenalectomy; bilateral hyperplasia → mineralocorticoid receptor antagonists (spironolactone 12.5–50 mg/day or eplerenone 25–50 mg BID). Monitor K⁺/Cr and BP.

2. Cushing: treat source (pituitary/ectopic/adrenal). Avoid empiric steroids for other conditions. Pre-op/bridge meds (ketoconazole, metyrapone, osilodrostat) are specialist-led.

3. PPGL: α-blockade FIRST (phenoxybenzamine or doxazosin) ± high-salt diet/volume repletion, then β-blocker if needed; definitive surgery. Avoid unopposed β-blockade.

4. PHPT: parathyroidectomy if surgical criteria met (symptoms, Ca >0.25 mmol/L [1 mg/dL] above ULN, osteoporosis/fragility fracture, nephrolithiasis/nephrocalcinosis, CrCl <60, age <50). Non-surgical: hydration, avoid thiazides/lithium; consider cinacalcet (specialist) and treat osteoporosis (bisphosphonates) if needed.

5. Primary Adrenal Insufficiency: hydrocortisone 15–25 mg/day in divided doses (or equivalent) + fludrocortisone 0.05–0.2 mg/day; sick-day rules; emergency IM hydrocortisone kit.

6. Hyperprolactinemia: dopamine agonists (cabergoline weekly or bromocriptine daily). Stop offending drugs if possible; treat hypothyroidism. Contraception/fertility counselling.

7. Acromegaly: transsphenoidal surgery is first-line; medical therapy (somatostatin analogues, GH receptor

antagonist, dopamine agonists) if persistent disease —
specialist-led.

C. PROCEDURES

1. Arrange appropriate imaging only AFTER biochemical
   confirmation (adrenal CT/MRI for PA/PPGL; pituitary
   MRI for prolactinomas/acromegaly; parathyroid
   imaging for surgical planning in PHPT).
2. Educate patients with AI on IM hydrocortisone use
   and provide medical alert identification; provide written
   sick-day plan.

DISPOSITION (DISCHARGE/OBSERVE/ TRANSFER) & RETURN PRECAUTIONS

1. Urgent ED/transfer: adrenal crisis (vomiting,
   hypotension, confusion), pheochromocytoma crisis
   (severe headache, diaphoresis, palpitations with
   HTN), severe hypercalcemia (confusion, dehydration,
   arrhythmia), pituitary apoplexy (sudden headache/
   vision loss).
2. Urgent endocrinology referral: positive screens for
   PA/Cushing/PPGL/PHPT/AI/hyperprolactinemia/
   acromegaly; symptomatic hypercalcemia; persistent
   unexplained resistant HTN.

PEARLS & PITFALLS

1. Screen PA in resistant HTN or HTN with hypokalemia
   — it's common and treatable; correct K^+ and review

meds before ARR.

2. Use ONE high-quality screen for Cushing; multiple positives reduce false positives; avoid testing during acute illness if possible.

3. Never start β-blocker before α-blocker in suspected PPGL.

4. High calcium with non-suppressed PTH = PHPT until proven otherwise; check vitamin D and urine calcium to exclude FHH.

5. Adrenal insufficiency: treat first (hydrocortisone), confirm later — don't delay if unstable.

REFERENCES

1. Endocrine Society Clinical Practice Guidelines (open summaries): Primary Aldosteronism (2016), Cushing Syndrome (2008/2015 update), Pheochromocytoma/ Paraganglioma (2014), Primary Adrenal Insufficiency (2016), Hyperprolactinemia (2011), Acromegaly (2014). endocrine.org

2. American Association of Clinical Endocrinology (AACE) / American Association of Endocrine Surgeons (AAES) public statements on Primary Hyperparathyroidism (open). aace.com / endocrine.org / endocrine surgery society sites

3. NICE Guidelines/CKS (open): Hypertension (secondary causes incl. PA), Hypercalcaemia/ Hyperparathyroidism, Adrenal insufficiency, Cushing's syndrome — topic pages. nice.org.uk / cks.nice.org.uk

4. AAFP. Practical reviews: Primary Aldosteronism; Hyperprolactinemia; Hypercalcemia; Diagnosis of Cushing Syndrome; Pheochromocytoma; Adrenal Insufficiency (open articles). aafp.org

5. Society for Endocrinology (UK). Emergency guidance: Adrenal crisis; patient resources for PPGL and PHPT (open). endocrinology.org

6. Cancer Research UK / NCI PDQ® (open): Pituitary tumours and adrenal tumours overviews relevant to endocrine disorders. cancerresearchuk.org / cancer. gov

THYROID DISEASES — HYPOTHYROIDISM & HYPERTHYROIDISM

OVERVIEW & "DON'T MISS"

1. Hypothyroidism: autoimmune (Hashimoto) most common; also post-radioiodine/surgery, drugs (amiodarone, lithium), iodine imbalance.

2. Hyperthyroidism: Graves disease, toxic multinodular goiter/adenoma, thyroiditis (painless/subacute), exogenous thyroid hormone.

3. DON'T MISS: myxedema coma (hypothermia, bradycardia, hypotension, AMS); thyroid storm (fever, tachyarrhythmia, delirium, heart failure); pregnancy-related complications; atrial fibrillation and osteoporosis from thyrotoxicosis.

HISTORY & EXAM

1. Hypo: fatigue, weight gain, cold intolerance, constipation, dry skin/hair loss, menorrhagia/infertility, depression; exam: bradycardia, delayed reflexes, goiter.

2. Hyper: weight loss, heat intolerance, palpitations/

tremor, anxiety, diarrhea, oligomenorrhea; exam: tachycardia/AF, tremor, proximal myopathy, lid lag; Graves ophthalmopathy/dermopathy in some.

3. Ask: meds (amiodarone, lithium, immune checkpoint inhibitors, interferon), iodine exposure/contrast, pregnancy/postpartum, family history, biotin use (assay interference).

DIFFERENTIAL DIAGNOSIS (TOP 5)

1. Subclinical hypo/hyperthyroidism (abnormal TSH with normal FT4).

2. Thyroiditis (painless/post-viral/subacute) with transient hyper → hypo → recovery.

3. Non-thyroidal illness (euthyroid sick syndrome).

4. Medication-induced (amiodarone, lithium, excess thyroid hormone).

5. Pituitary/hypothalamic disease (central hypo/hyper — discordant TSH/FT4).

INVESTIGATIONS (POC/LABS/IMAGING)

1. First-line: TSH. If abnormal or high suspicion, add free T4 (± total/FT3 if hyper suspected or T3-predominant).

2. Autoantibodies: anti-TPO (hypo/Hashimoto), TSI/TRAb (Graves).

3. If low TSH with high FT4/FT3: differentiate increased synthesis vs. release/factitious — consider radioactive iodine uptake (contraindicated in pregnancy) or TRAb; ESR/CRP elevated in subacute thyroiditis.

4. Ultrasound: only if palpable nodule/asymmetry/goiter; not routine for biochemical disease.

5. Baseline before antithyroid drugs: CBC and liver enzymes. ECG if tachyarrhythmia; pregnancy test in reproductive-potential patients before radioiodine/ ATDs.

MANAGEMENT (NON-PHARM → MEDS → PROCEDURES)

A. NON-PHARMACOLOGIC

1. Education: timing and interactions (e.g., levothyroxine on empty stomach; separate from iron/calcium by ≥4 hours).

2. Stop biotin 48–72 h before thyroid labs to avoid assay interference.

3. Smoking cessation (worsens Graves ophthalmopathy); selenium-adequate diet may support thyroiditis recovery (evidence mixed).

B. MEDICATIONS (EXAMPLES; INDIVIDUALIZE)

1. Hypothyroidism (primary): levothyroxine ~1.6 mcg/ kg/day for healthy adults <60 without CVD; start lower (12.5–25 mcg/day) in elderly/CVD, titrate q6–8 weeks to normalize TSH. Aim upper-normal FT4 in pregnancy; increase dose by ~25–30% once pregnancy confirmed (e.g., +2 extra tablets/week).

2. Subclinical hypothyroidism: consider treatment if TSH ≥10 mIU/L, or TSH 4.5–9.9 with symptoms, positive

TPOAb, goiter, pregnancy/infertility, or CVD risk —
shared decision-making.

3. Hyperthyroidism (symptom control): non-selective
   beta-blocker e.g., propranolol 10–40 mg q6–8h (or
   LA), or atenolol/metoprolol if contraindications to
   propranolol.

4. Antithyroid drugs (ATDs): methimazole (first-line
   except 1st trimester/thyroid storm) initial 10–30 mg
   daily; adjust to keep FT4 near normal. PTU reserved
   for 1st trimester or storm (e.g., 50–150 mg TID;
   monitor hepatotoxicity). Educate re agranulocytosis/
   hepatitis (stop and check if fever, sore throat,
   jaundice).

5. Graves options: ATDs for 12–18 months with remission
   attempt vs. radioiodine ablation vs. thyroidectomy —
   consider age, goiter size, ophthalmopathy, pregnancy
   plans.

6. Thyroiditis (subacute/painless): ATDs not indicated
   (hormone leakage). Use NSAIDs; if severe pain or
   persistent, prednisone 40 mg daily taper over 2–4
   weeks; beta-blocker for symptoms.

7. Thyroid storm: emergency — ICU, PTU loading
   500–1000 mg then 250 mg q4h, iodine 1 h after PTU,
   beta-blocker, hydrocortisone 100 mg q8h, supportive
   care (follow institutional protocol).

8. Myxedema coma: emergency — ICU, IV levothyroxine
   ± liothyronine per protocol, hydrocortisone until
   adrenal insufficiency excluded, active warming and
   supportive care.

C. PROCEDURES

1. Radioiodine ablation for Graves/toxic nodular disease when indicated (contraindicated in pregnancy/ breastfeeding).

2. Thyroidectomy for very large goiters, compressive symptoms, suspicious nodules, or patient preference/ intolerance to other therapies.

3. Nodule evaluation with FNA follows standard risk-stratified ultrasound criteria (beyond scope).

DISPOSITION (DISCHARGE/OBSERVE/ TRANSFER) & RETURN PRECAUTIONS

1. Discharge most stable outpatients with clear plan: labs in 6–8 weeks after any dose change (hypo) or q4–6 weeks while titrating ATDs (hyper).

2. Urgent same-day/ED: suspected thyroid storm or myxedema coma; severe tachyarrhythmia/heart failure; chest pain/ACS; pregnancy with severe hyper/ hypothyroidism; compressive goiter with stridor.

3. Return immediately for: fever/sore throat (possible agranulocytosis on ATDs), jaundice/dark urine, palpitations/syncope, progressive dyspnea/stridor, or new neurologic changes.

PEARLS & PITFALLS

1. Take levothyroxine consistently (same time/brand); separate from calcium/iron/PPIs; consider bedtime dosing if mornings challenging.

2. Check for adrenal insufficiency if clinical clues before starting thyroid hormone in severe hypothyroidism.

3. In pregnancy: PTU in 1st trimester, switch to methimazole thereafter; aim FT4 high-normal; avoid radioiodine.

4. Subclinical hyperthyroidism (TSH <0.1) in older adults or with AF/osteoporosis warrants treatment consideration.

5. Smoking cessation and local measures for mild Graves eye disease; refer to ophthalmology for moderate–severe cases.

REFERENCES

1. NICE Clinical Knowledge Summaries (CKS). Hypothyroidism; Thyrotoxicosis/Hyperthyroidism — open access guidance. cks.nice.org.uk

2. American Thyroid Association (ATA). Hyperthyroidism and other causes of thyrotoxicosis: management guidelines (open summaries) & patient resources. thyroid.org

3. Endotext (NCBI Bookshelf). Hypothyroidism in Adults; Graves' Disease & other thyrotoxicosis chapters — open access. ncbi.nlm.nih.gov/books

4. AAFP. Hypothyroidism: Diagnosis and Treatment; Hyperthyroidism: Diagnosis and Treatment — open articles. aafp.org

5. BC Guidelines. Thyroid Function Testing & Hypothyroidism/Hyperthyroidism primary care

pathways (public). bcguidelines.gov.bc.ca

6. StatPearls (NCBI). Thyroid Storm; Myxedema Coma — open access clinical reviews. ncbi.nlm.nih.gov/books

7. Choosing Wisely Canada. Thyroid testing/management recommendations (public). choosingwiselycanada.org

THYROID NODULE

OVERVIEW & "DON'T MISS"

1. Very common; most are benign. Aim: identify nodules needing biopsy/surgery vs. safe surveillance.

2. Cancer risk overall ~5–10% (higher with suspicious ultrasound/LN).

3. DON'T MISS: rapidly enlarging mass, stridor/airway compromise, hoarseness (recurrent laryngeal nerve), hard fixed nodule or abnormal cervical lymph nodes, prior childhood head/neck irradiation, family history of medullary thyroid cancer/MEN2, pregnancy with severe compressive symptoms.

HISTORY & EXAM

1. Symptoms: growth, neck pressure, dysphagia, dyspnea when supine, hoarseness, pain (subacute thyroiditis).

2. Risk factors: childhood radiation exposure; nuclear fallout exposure; family history (thyroid cancer, MEN2); age <20 or >60; male sex. Iodine deficiency regions; autoimmune thyroid disease.

3. Meds/exposures: amiodarone, lithium; biotin use (lab

interference); pregnancy/postpartum.

4. Exam: nodule size/consistency/fixation; thyroid tenderness; complete cervical lymph node exam; voice changes.

DIFFERENTIAL DIAGNOSIS (TOP 5)

1. Benign colloid nodule / multinodular goiter.

2. Thyroid cyst (simple or complex).

3. Thyroiditis-related 'pseudonodule' (painless/subacute).

4. Follicular neoplasm (adenoma vs. carcinoma — FNA cannot assess capsular/vascular invasion).

5. Papillary or medullary thyroid carcinoma (± metastatic nodes).

INVESTIGATIONS (POC/LABS/IMAGING)

1. TSH first-line. If low/suppressed → assess for hyperfunctioning ('hot') nodule with radionuclide uptake scan (I-123 preferred). Hot nodules are rarely malignant — FNA usually not indicated.

2. High-resolution thyroid + cervical lymph node ultrasound for ALL nodules to risk-stratify (hypoechoic, microcalcifications, irregular/lobulated margins, taller-than-wide, extrathyroidal extension; benign: spongiform, purely cystic).

3. Use a structured system (e.g., ACR TI-RADS 2017) to guide FNA and follow-up:

4. TR3: follow-up if ≥1.5 cm; FNA if ≥2.5 cm. • TR4: follow-up if ≥1.0 cm; FNA if ≥1.5 cm. • TR5: follow-up if

≥0.5 cm; FNA if ≥1.0 cm. (TR1–2: no FNA).

5. Alternate (ATA 2015): high/intermediate-suspicion ≥1 cm; low-suspicion ≥1.5 cm; very-low suspicion consider ≥2 cm.

6. FNA cytology reported by Bethesda System (I–VI) with corresponding malignancy risks and management; repeat FNA for nondiagnostic (I).

7. Consider calcitonin if MTC suspected (family history, suspicious LN, diarrhea/flushing); not routine screening. Do not order Tg for diagnosis.

8. Laryngoscopy if hoarseness persists or pre-op; pregnancy test when appropriate.

MANAGEMENT (NON-PHARM → MEDS → PROCEDURES)

A. NON-PHARMACOLOGIC

1. Reassurance + surveillance for benign, low-risk nodules using US intervals (see below).

2. Avoid empiric levothyroxine 'suppression therapy' for benign nodules — limited benefit, risk of subclinical hyperthyroidism (AF, bone loss).

3. Iodine adequacy via balanced diet; counsel on biotin stopping 48–72 h before thyroid labs.

B. MEDICATIONS (EXAMPLES; INDIVIDUALIZE)

1. Toxic ('hot') nodule causing hyperthyroidism: beta-blocker for symptoms; methimazole as bridge;

definitive therapy with radioiodine ablation or surgery (radioiodine contraindicated in pregnancy).

2. Subacute thyroiditis nodules: NSAIDs; short prednisone taper if severe; beta-blocker for thyrotoxic symptoms. Antithyroid drugs are NOT indicated for thyroiditis.

C. PROCEDURES

1. Ultrasound-guided FNA per risk/size thresholds; repeat FNA if nondiagnostic or if growth/new suspicious features.

2. Benign symptomatic nodules: consider surgical hemithyroidectomy vs. minimally invasive ablation (ethanol ablation for recurrent cysts; radiofrequency/ laser ablation where available).

3. Suspicious/malignant cytology (Bethesda V–VI) or follicular neoplasm (IV): endocrine surgery referral; consider hemithyroidectomy vs. total thyroidectomy per guideline and tumor factors.

DISPOSITION (DISCHARGE/OBSERVE/ TRANSFER) & RETURN PRECAUTIONS

1. Discharge most with plan: surveillance ultrasound intervals (e.g., ACR TI-RADS suggested: TR3 at 1, 3, 5 years; TR4 at 1, 2, 3, 5; TR5 yearly up to 5).

2. Observe/urgent review: rapid growth, new hoarseness, compressive symptoms, or suspicious lymph nodes.

3. Refer: Bethesda III–VI cytology; abnormal cervical

nodes; toxic nodule for definitive therapy; pregnancy with significant compressive symptoms.

4. Return immediately for: progressive dyspnea/stridor, dysphagia with aspiration, voice change, or acute swelling/pain.

PEARLS & PITFALLS

1. Hyperfunctioning ('hot') nodules are rarely malignant — prioritize treating hyperthyroidism rather than FNA.

2. Ultrasound features drive decision-making more than size alone; document TI-RADS/ATA category in notes.

3. Meaningful growth: ≥20% increase in at least two dimensions (≥2 mm) or volume increase >50% — consider repeat FNA if new suspicious features accompany growth.

4. Do not routinely ultrasound patients with abnormal TSH but no palpable nodule (Choosing Wisely).

5. Pregnancy: FNA is safe; defer radioiodine; surgery only for compelling indications (2nd trimester if needed).

REFERENCES

1. Haugen BR, et al. 2015 American Thyroid Association Management Guidelines for Adult Patients with Thyroid Nodules and Differentiated Thyroid Cancer. (Open access via PubMed Central).

2. American College of Radiology (ACR) TI-RADS (2017) — White paper & public summaries of scoring and

thresholds.

3. NICE Guideline NG145. Thyroid disease: assessment and management (2019, updates online).

4. Endotext (NCBI Bookshelf). Thyroid Nodule — Evaluation and Management (open access).

5. AAFP. Thyroid Nodules: Advances in Evaluation and Management (open article).

6. Choosing Wisely Canada. Thyroid ultrasound and testing recommendations (public).

7. BC Guidelines. Thyroid Function Testing & Thyroid Nodule pathways (public).

OBESITY — FAMILY MEDICINE OFFICE

OVERVIEW & "DON'T MISS"

1. Chronic, relapsing disease of abnormal or excess adiposity with health risk; management = long-term, multi-component (nutrition, physical activity, behavior, medications, and procedures).

2. Classify risk beyond BMI: add waist circumference (central adiposity), complications (T2D, HTN, ASCVD, OSA, NAFLD/MASLD, OA, GERD, infertility).

3. Typical initial target: ≥5–10% weight loss at 3–6 months; reassess and escalate if <5% with good adherence.

4. DON'T MISS: secondary/endocrine causes (Cushing, hypothyroidism, hypogonadism), medication-induced weight gain (antipsychotics, valproate, TCAs/SSRIs, insulin/sulfonylureas, β-blockers, corticosteroids, progestins), eating disorders (binge eating, bulimia), OSA/OHS, pregnancy, depression/suicidality.

HISTORY & EXAM

1. Weight timeline (highest/lowest), prior attempts and responses, triggers, night eating/binge patterns, shift

work, sleep, mood, stress, trauma/abuse history (ACE).

2. Dietary recall (24-h + typical week), beverages/alcohol; activity/sedentary time; readiness/goal setting; social supports; financial/food access.

3. Medications causing gain; reproductive history (PCOS, fertility, contraception, pregnancy plan).

4. Exam: BP, BMI, waist circumference; signs of endocrine disease (striae, bruising, proximal weakness), hirsutism/acanthosis; joint pain/gait; airway/mallampati (OSA).

DIFFERENTIAL DIAGNOSIS (TOP 5)

1. Primary (polygenic) obesity with lifestyle/environmental drivers.

2. Medication-induced weight gain (antipsychotics, insulin/SU, valproate, mirtazapine, steroids).

3. Endocrine: hypothyroidism, Cushing syndrome, hypogonadism, PCOS.

4. Hypothalamic/pituitary disease; rare genetic syndromes (e.g., leptin–melanocortin pathway).

5. Fluid retention/edema or organomegaly mimicking weight gain.

INVESTIGATIONS (POC/LABS/IMAGING)

1. Baseline labs (tailor): A1C or fasting glucose; fasting lipid panel; ALT/AST (MASLD screen); TSH if symptoms/risk; creatinine/eGFR; consider urine ACR

(if diabetes/HTN).

2. Screen complications: STOP-Bang for OSA; BP; consider NAFLD fibrosis score/FIB-4 if elevated ALT or metabolic risk; depression/anxiety screen (PHQ-9/ GAD-7).

3. Pregnancy test before starting weight-loss medications contraindicated in pregnancy; baseline weight/waist for monitoring.

MANAGEMENT (NON-PHARM → MEDS → PROCEDURES)

A. NON-PHARMACOLOGIC (FIRST-LINE FOR ALL)

1. Behavioral treatment (≥12 sessions in 6 mo if possible): goal-setting, self-monitoring (logs/CGM-style feedback), stimulus control, problem-solving, relapse prevention, motivational interviewing.

2. Nutrition: create energy deficit (e.g., −500 to −750 kcal/ day) with patient-preferred pattern (Mediterranean, DASH, low-carb, high-protein, meal-replacement), high protein (≈1.0–1.2 g/kg/day) to preserve lean mass unless contraindicated.

3. Physical activity: ≥150 min/wk moderate + 2–3×/wk resistance; more (200–300 min/wk) to maintain loss; start low, progress gradually; reduce sedentary time.

4. Sleep & mental health: treat OSA; optimize sleep hygiene (7–9 h); address depression, binge eating; consider therapy referral.

5. Med review: substitute weight-neutral/-reducing alternatives when feasible (e.g., switch SGAs, use GLP-1/SGLT2 in T2D).

B. MEDICATIONS FOR CHRONIC WEIGHT MANAGEMENT (EXAMPLES; CHECK LABELS/ ELIGIBILITY)

1. Indications (adults): BMI ≥30, or ≥27 with ≥1 weight-related comorbidity (T2D, HTN, dyslipidemia, OSA, etc.), as adjunct to lifestyle.

2. GLP-1 receptor agonist — semaglutide 2.4 mg SC weekly (titrate over 16–20 wks): high efficacy; GI effects; avoid in personal/family MTC/MEN2; monitor gallbladder/pancreatitis risk.

3. Dual GIP/GLP-1 agonist — tirzepatide SC weekly (titrate): very high efficacy; similar GI precautions; avoid in MTC/MEN2; monitor for hypoglycemia if used with insulin/SU in diabetes.

4. Liraglutide 3.0 mg SC daily: moderate efficacy; GI effects; MTC/MEN2 warning.

5. Phentermine/topiramate ER PO daily: moderate–high efficacy; teratogenic — mandatory contraception & monthly pregnancy tests; avoid in uncontrolled HTN/ CAD; monitor mood/cognition.

6. Naltrexone/bupropion ER PO: moderate efficacy; avoid in seizure disorder, uncontrolled HTN, chronic opioid therapy, eating disorders; monitor mood/suicidality; nausea common.

7. Orlistat PO TID with fat-containing meals: modest

efficacy; GI side effects; supplement fat-soluble vitamins.

8. Set realistic expectations: if <5% loss after 12–16 weeks at therapeutic dose, discontinue or switch; combine with lifestyle and consider escalation.

C. PROCEDURES (METABOLIC/BARIATRIC & ENDOSCOPIC)

1. Surgery indications (ASMBS/IFSO 2022): BMI ≥35 regardless of comorbidities; consider BMI 30–34.9 with metabolic disease not controlled by medical therapy; lower BMI thresholds for Asian ancestry may apply. Refer to experienced center.

2. Common procedures: sleeve gastrectomy; Roux-en-Y gastric bypass (RYGB). Benefits: largest, durable loss and comorbidity improvement (T2D, OSA, HTN).

3. Endoscopic options (availability varies): intragastric balloon (temporary), endoscopic sleeve gastroplasty — consider for BMI 30–40 when surgery is declined/ inappropriate.

4. Peri-/post-op care: micronutrient supplementation (multivitamin + B12 + iron + calcium/vit D), pregnancy avoidance 12–18 months post-op, hypoglycemia monitoring in diabetes, lifelong follow-up.

DISPOSITION (DISCHARGE/OBSERVE/ TRANSFER) & RETURN PRECAUTIONS

1. Outpatient management for most; schedule follow-up

q4–12 weeks during active titration, then q3–6 months.

2. Urgent care/ED: severe abdominal pain/persistent vomiting on GLP-1 (rule out gallstones/pancreatitis), chest pain/palpitations on sympathomimetic agents, suicidal ideation on naltrexone/bupropion, post-op complications (bleeding, leak, obstruction).

3. Return if weight ↑ >3% from nadir, medication intolerance, recurrent hypoglycemia (if diabetes meds), or pregnancy planning.

PEARLS & PITFALLS

1. Use complication-centric staging (e.g., Edmonton Obesity Staging System) to prioritize therapy intensity.

2. Avoid weight-loss pharmacotherapy in pregnancy/ breastfeeding; stop 2 months before planned conception for agents with long washout (e.g., semaglutide/tirzepatide).

3. For steroid bursts or atypical antipsychotics, pre-empt with nutrition/activity plan and consider agents with weight benefit (e.g., metformin for SGA-associated gain).

4. Expect weight regain after stopping meds — plan for long-term therapy when effective and tolerated.

5. After bariatric surgery, avoid NSAIDs (RYGB ulcer risk) and monitor for alcohol misuse transfer.

REFERENCES

1. NICE Guideline NG7. Obesity: identification,

assessment and management (public). nice.org.uk

2. AGA Clinical Practice Guideline on Pharmacological Interventions for Adults with Obesity (open access 2022). gastro.org & journals.gastro.org

3. Obesity Canada. Clinical Practice Guidelines (open access). obesitycanada.ca

4. WHO. Obesity and Overweight — Fact sheet & guidelines (public). who.int

5. CDC. Adult Obesity Causes & Consequences; Lifestyle resources (public). cdc.gov

6. ASMBS/IFSO 2022 Guidelines: Indications for Metabolic and Bariatric Surgery (open PDF). asmbs. org

7. Diabetes Canada / ADA open resources on obesity in diabetes and GLP-1/GIP agents (public summaries). diabetes.ca / diabetesjournals.org

RENAL & UROLOGY
(ADULT MALE HEALTH)

NEPHROLITHIASIS (KIDNEY STONES)

OVERVIEW & "DON'T MISS"

1. Typical: sudden colicky flank pain radiating to groin/ testicle/labia ± N/V, hematuria. Most stones are calcium oxalate; others: uric acid, struvite, cystine.

2. DON'T MISS: infected obstructing stone (fever, rigors, toxic, pyuria/positive culture) → emergent urologic decompression; anuria/solitary kidney/bilateral obstruction; pregnancy; AKI; uncontrolled pain/ vomiting; AAA in older patients with back/abdo pain.

HISTORY & EXAM

1. History: onset, colicky pattern, radiation, hematuria, dysuria, fever/chills, prior stones, anatomic disease, recent dehydration, gout, bariatric/IBD, diet (salt, oxalate, animal protein), medications (topiramate, acetazolamide, indinavir, loop diuretics, vitamin C).

2. Exam: vitals (fever, tachycardia), CVA tenderness, abdominal exam, hydration status; pelvic/testicular exam when indicated; septic signs.

DIFFERENTIAL DIAGNOSIS (TOP 5)

1. Pyelonephritis/UTI with or without obstruction.

2. AAA/renal infarct (vascular): consider in older patients or atypical pain.

3. Appendicitis, biliary/peptic disease (epigastric/RUQ), bowel obstruction.

4. Gynecologic: ectopic pregnancy, ovarian torsion, ruptured cyst.

5. Genitourinary: testicular torsion, epididymo-orchitis.

INVESTIGATIONS (POC/LABS/IMAGING)

1. POC: urinalysis with microscopy (hematuria, WBCs, nitrites, crystals); urine culture if infection suspected; urine pregnancy test in reproductive-potential patients.

2. Labs: CBC if febrile/systemic; creatinine/eGFR, electrolytes; CRP if infection concern.

3. Imaging: ultrasound first in pregnancy and many young/low-risk; assesses hydronephrosis. Non-contrast low-dose CT KUB is most sensitive/ specific for adults with uncertain diagnosis or complications. KUB X-ray has limited value (radiolucent uric acid, many non-visible).

4. Consider POCUS for hydronephrosis if available; avoid contrast CT for stones unless alternative Dx sought.

MANAGEMENT (NON-PHARM → MEDS → PROCEDURES)

A. NON-PHARMACOLOGIC

1. Analgesia and antiemetics promptly; encourage oral fluids as tolerated (no forced diuresis).
2. Strain urine to capture stone for analysis; activity as tolerated.
3. Counsel red flags (fever, anuria, uncontrolled pain/ vomiting).

B. MEDICATIONS (EXAMPLES; INDIVIDUALIZE)

1. Pain: NSAIDs first-line if renal function adequate (e.g., ketorolac 10–30 mg PO/IM; ibuprofen/naproxen scheduled). Opioid adjunct if refractory.
2. Antiemetics (ondansetron, metoclopramide) PRN.
3. Medical expulsive therapy (MET): tamsulosin 0.4 mg HS up to 4–6 weeks can improve passage for distal ureteral stones ~5–10 mm; limited benefit for very small/large stones.
4. Antibiotics if UTI evidence or sepsis; tailor to culture; avoid delaying decompression in infected obstruction.

C. PROCEDURES

1. Urgent urology for decompression (ureteral stent or percutaneous nephrostomy) if infected obstruction, anuria/solitary kidney, worsening AKI, uncontrolled pain/vomiting, pregnancy with obstruction, or failure of

outpatient management.

2. Elective: ESWL, ureteroscopy (URS), or PCNL depending on size/location and patient factors (typically ≥10 mm, proximal location, or persistent obstruction).

DISPOSITION (DISCHARGE/OBSERVE/ TRANSFER) & RETURN PRECAUTIONS

1. Discharge: afebrile, pain/nausea controlled with oral meds, stable renal function, small stone likely to pass, reliable follow-up within 1–2 weeks.

2. Observe/same-day reassessment: diagnostic uncertainty, moderate hydronephrosis with stable vitals, social barriers, or inadequate pain control.

3. Transfer/Admit: suspected infected obstruction, sepsis, AKI, solitary kidney/bilateral obstruction, pregnancy with obstruction, or uncontrolled symptoms.

4. Return immediately for: fever/chills, worsening pain, persistent vomiting, anuria, fainting, or new weakness/ numbness.

PEARLS & PITFALLS

1. NSAIDs are superior to opioids for renal colic and reduce ureteral smooth-muscle spasm.

2. CT sensitivity is high, but ultrasound first avoids radiation in pregnancy/younger patients; correlate with clinical suspicion.

3. Do not delay source control for infected obstruction — antibiotics alone are insufficient.

4. Recurrent/high-risk stone formers: encourage urine output ≥2–2.5 L/day; reduce sodium; moderate animal protein; maintain normal dietary calcium with meals; limit high-oxalate foods; add citrate (citrus) intake.

5. After a stone event or in recurrent cases, consider metabolic work-up (24-h urine, serum Ca, PTH if hypercalcemia) and targeted prevention (e.g., thiazides, potassium citrate, allopurinol) guided by results.

REFERENCES

1. NICE Guideline NG118. Renal and ureteric stones: assessment and management (public). nice.org.uk

2. Canadian Urological Association (CUA). Guideline on the evaluation and medical management of kidney stones (open access). cuaj.ca

3. American Urological Association (AUA). Medical management of kidney stones (summary statements available publicly). auanet.org

4. Emergency Care BC. Renal Colic — Clinical Summary (public). emergencycarebc.ca

5. Merck Manual Professional. Nephrolithiasis — evaluation & management (open). merckmanuals.com

6. National Kidney Foundation (NKF). Kidney Stones patient/provider resources (public). kidney.org

7. Choosing Wisely Canada. Imaging for renal colic recommendations (public). choosingwiselycanada.org

UTI / PYELONEPHRITIS & PROSTATITIS (RE-GEN)

OVERVIEW & "DON'T MISS"

1. Spectrum from uncomplicated cystitis → complicated UTI → pyelonephritis/urosepsis. Men and pregnancy are complicated by definition.

2. DON'T MISS: obstructed infected stone (fever + flank pain + hydronephrosis) → emergent decompression; sepsis; pregnancy with pyelo (usually admit). Consider STI (urethritis/cervicitis) in dysuria without pyuria.

HISTORY & EXAM

1. Cystitis: dysuria, frequency, urgency, suprapubic pain, new hematuria; no vaginal discharge.

2. Pyelonephritis: fever, flank pain, chills, N/V, CVA tenderness.

3. Prostatitis: perineal/suprapubic pain, dysuria, obstructive LUTS, painful ejaculation, fever/chills; avoid vigorous prostate massage.

4. Risk: pregnancy, male, catheter, recent antibiotics, diabetes, urologic anomalies, nephrolithiasis, MSM/

new partner.

5. Exam: vitals; CVA tenderness; abdominal/suprapubic tenderness; targeted GU exam; gentle DRE (boggy/tender prostate suggests acute bacterial prostatitis).

DIFFERENTIAL DIAGNOSIS (TOP 5)

1. Urethritis/cervicitis (chlamydia/gonorrhea/trichomonas).

2. Vaginitis (BV/candida/trichomonas).

3. Nephrolithiasis/obstruction.

4. Appendicitis/gynecologic causes (ectopic, torsion).

5. BPH/retention; bladder pain syndrome.

INVESTIGATIONS (POC/LABS/IMAGING)

1. UA with microscopy; urine culture before antibiotics when feasible (always for pyelo, men, pregnancy, recurrent/complicated).

2. Pregnancy test for those with reproductive potential.

3. STI NAAT when urethral discharge, dysuria without pyuria, or risk factors.

4. Pyelo/severe: CBC, creatinine/eGFR, electrolytes; blood cultures if febrile/rigors; lactate if septic.

5. Imaging: none for simple cystitis. Renal US or non-contrast CT if obstruction suspected, atypical course, or no improvement in 48–72 h. POCUS for hydronephrosis if available.

6. Prostatitis: UA/culture; avoid PSA in acute infection; check PVR if retention.

MANAGEMENT (NON-PHARM → MEDS → PROCEDURES)

A. NON-PHARMACOLOGIC

1. Hydration as tolerated; analgesia/antipyretics; phenazopyridine 200 mg PO TID × ≤2 days for dysuria (avoid in G6PD).

2. Catheter-associated: remove/replace catheter; culture from new catheter before antibiotics.

3. Education: adherence, hydration, post-coital voiding (limited evidence), red-flag symptoms, and follow-up plan.

B. MEDICATIONS (EXAMPLES; TAILOR TO LOCAL RESISTANCE, ALLERGIES, PREGNANCY)

1. Uncomplicated cystitis (non-pregnant adult): nitrofurantoin 100 mg BID × 5 days; TMP-SMX 160/800 mg BID × 3 days if local resistance <20%; fosfomycin 3 g once. Avoid FQs for simple cystitis.

2. Complicated cystitis / male lower UTI: 5–7 (up to 14) days depending on agent/response. Nitrofurantoin is bladder-only (not for pyelo). Oral β-lactams (e.g., amox-clav, cephalexin) are options if susceptible.

3. Acute pyelonephritis (outpatient): ciprofloxacin 500 mg BID × 7 days (or 1000 mg ER × 7) OR levofloxacin 750 mg daily × 5; OR TMP-SMX BID × 14 if susceptible. Consider one dose ceftriaxone 1 g IM/IV (or gentamicin) if resistance likely.

4. Acute pyelonephritis (inpatient/severe): IV ceftriaxone ± aminoglycoside, or piperacillin-tazobactam for severe sepsis; step-down to oral to complete 7–14 days total.

5. Pregnancy (ASB or cystitis): 4–7 days cephalexin, amox-clav, or nitrofurantoin (avoid near term); fosfomycin 3 g once is an option. Avoid FQs; avoid TMP-SMX in 1st trimester and near term. Do test-of-cure culture 1–2 weeks after therapy.

6. Acute bacterial prostatitis: ciprofloxacin 500 mg BID or levofloxacin 500–750 mg daily OR TMP-SMX BID for 2–4 weeks; admit for sepsis/retention/comorbidity. Add α-blocker (tamsulosin). Prefer suprapubic catheter over urethral if retention.

7. Chronic bacterial prostatitis: 4–6 weeks FQ or TMP-SMX per culture; consider urology referral. CP/CPPS: multimodal (α-blocker, NSAIDs, pelvic floor physio, neuropathic pain agents).

C. PROCEDURES

1. Urgent urology for obstructed infected stone (stent or nephrostomy).

2. Bladder drainage for acute urinary retention (consider suprapubic catheter in severe prostatitis).

DISPOSITION (DISCHARGE/OBSERVE/TRANSFER) & RETURN PRECAUTIONS

1. Discharge: improving, able to take PO, pain controlled,

reliable follow-up at 48–72 h; provide written precautions.

2. Observe/same-day: persistent vomiting, frailty, diagnostic uncertainty, or inadequate supports; pregnancy with pyelo usually admit.

3. Admit/Transfer: sepsis, obstruction, pregnancy with pyelo, immunocompromise, severe comorbidity, failure of outpatient therapy, urinary retention needing drainage.

4. Return immediately: fever/rigors, increasing flank pain, anuria, confusion, chest pain/SOB, or worse after 24–48 h of antibiotics.

PEARLS & PITFALLS

1. Do NOT use nitrofurantoin or fosfomycin for pyelonephritis (poor tissue penetration).

2. Consider STI when dysuria without pyuria or with urethral discharge.

3. Screen/treat asymptomatic bacteriuria only in pregnancy or prior to certain urologic procedures.

4. Avoid PSA in acute prostatitis (false elevation).

5. Reassess at 48–72 h — lack of improvement → review culture/antibiogram and image for obstruction.

REFERENCES

1. IDSA — Acute Uncomplicated Cystitis & Pyelonephritis; Catheter-associated UTI; Asymptomatic Bacteriuria (open access). idsociety.org

2. NICE NG109 (Lower UTI) & NG111 (Pyelonephritis) — adults. nice.org.uk

3. BC Guidelines — Urinary Tract Infections (adults) & Pyelonephritis (public). bcguidelines.gov.bc.ca

4. Emergency Care BC — Pyelonephritis; UTI; Prostatitis summaries. emergencycarebc.ca

5. Canadian Urological Association — prostatitis/UTI resources (open). cuaj.ca

6. AAFP / Merck Manual — open clinical reviews. aafp.org / merckmanuals.com

7. PHAC — Antimicrobial stewardship & pregnancy safety resources. canada.ca

BPH/URINARY RETENTION • PROSTATITIS • PROSTATE CANCER

OVERVIEW & "DON'T MISS"

1. Lower urinary tract symptoms (LUTS) in men commonly due to benign prostatic hyperplasia (BPH), infection/inflammation, medications, or malignancy.

2. DON'T MISS: acute urinary retention (AUR) with obstructive uropathy, urosepsis from acute bacterial prostatitis, epididymo-orchitis/abscess, urinary retention from neurologic emergency (cauda equina), gross hematuria with clots/obstruction, prostate cancer with bone pain/weight loss.

HISTORY & EXAM

1. LUTS detail: voiding (weak stream, hesitancy, straining, intermittency, incomplete emptying) vs storage (frequency, urgency, nocturia, incontinence).

2. Screen red flags: fever/chills, dysuria, flank pain, hematuria (gross/microscopic), urinary retention, back pain/neurologic deficits, weight loss, bone pain.

3. Prostatitis clues: acute pelvic/perineal pain, dysuria,

obstructive symptoms, tender/boggy prostate (avoid vigorous DRE in suspected acute bacterial prostatitis).

4. Medications: anticholinergics (TCAs, oxybutynin), antihistamines, decongestants (α-agonists), opioids, benzodiazepines; alcohol; caffeine.

5. Exam: vitals; abdominal palpation/percussion for distended bladder; DRE (size/consistency, nodules/asymmetry, tenderness); focused neuro exam (saddle anesthesia, leg weakness).

DIFFERENTIAL DIAGNOSIS (TOP 5)

1. BPH/LUTS due to benign prostatic enlargement or bladder dysfunction.

2. Acute/chronic bacterial prostatitis; chronic pelvic pain syndrome.

3. UTI, urethritis, epididymo-orchitis; bladder stones.

4. Medication-induced urinary retention; neurogenic bladder (DM, MS, spinal stenosis/cauda equina).

5. Prostate cancer; less often bladder cancer (esp. with hematuria/smoking).

INVESTIGATIONS (POC/LABS/IMAGING)

1. Urinalysis ± culture for LUTS/UTI symptoms; consider STI NAAT if urethritis risk.

2. PSA: use shared decision-making (see below). Avoid PSA during acute prostatitis, UTI, urinary retention, or soon after instrumentation/ejaculation; recheck ≥6–8 weeks after resolution. 5-ARIs lower PSA ~50% after

6+ months (double measured value for interpretation).

3. Post-void residual (PVR) by bladder scan if retention/overflow suspected; >200 mL suggests significant retention.

4. CBC, creatinine if infection/systemic illness or suspected obstructive uropathy. Ultrasound kidneys/bladder if recurrent retention, hematuria, or renal insufficiency.

5. For prostate cancer suspicion (abnormal DRE or elevated PSA) → urology referral (MRI-guided risk assessment/biopsy per specialist).

MANAGEMENT (NON-PHARM → MEDS → PROCEDURES)

A. BPH/LUTS & URINARY RETENTION

1. Lifestyle: reduce evening fluids/caffeine/alcohol; timed voiding; treat constipation; review/stop offending meds.

2. α-blockers (first-line for moderate–severe bothersome LUTS): tamsulosin 0.4 mg HS, alfuzosin 10 mg daily, silodosin 8 mg daily, doxazosin/terazosin (titrate) — counsel on dizziness/retrograde ejaculation.

3. 5-α-reductase inhibitors (enlarged prostate/PSA ≥1.5 ng/mL or prostate ☐40 mL): finasteride 5 mg daily or dutasteride 0.5 mg daily; slower onset (6–12 mo), reduce AUR/surgery risk.

4. Combination α-blocker + 5-ARI for large prostates/high progression risk. Tadalafil 5 mg daily helps LUTS

± ED.

5. Storage-predominant symptoms with low PVR: add antimuscarinic (e.g., solifenacin) or β3-agonist (mirabegron). Avoid antimuscarinics in high PVR/ retention risk.

6. Acute urinary retention: immediate bladder decompression (urethral catheter; suprapubic if difficult). Start α-blocker and attempt trial without catheter (TWOC) in ~3–7 days. Evaluate precipitants (meds, constipation, infection, postoperative). Recurrent retention/renal insufficiency → urology.

7. Surgery indications (refer): refractory retention, recurrent UTIs, bladder stones, recurrent gross hematuria due to BPH, renal insufficiency from BOO, or persistent severe LUTS despite meds. Options include TURP/HoLEP, minimally invasive (Rezūm, UroLift) — specialist-led.

B. PROSTATITIS

1. Acute bacterial prostatitis (ABP): systemic features common. Avoid prostatic massage. If toxic/urinary retention/pyelonephritis → ED for IV antibiotics and possible drainage.

2. Outpatient ABP (mild-moderate, low resistance risk): culture-guided therapy; options include levofloxacin 500–750 mg daily or ciprofloxacin 500 mg BID, OR TMP-SMX DS BID if susceptible; typical duration 2–4 weeks. Provide analgesia, hydration, stool softener.

3. If STI suspected (younger, urethritis): ceftriaxone 500

mg IM once (1 g if ≥150 kg) + doxycycline 100 mg BID × 14 days; extend/modify per cultures and clinical course.

4. Chronic bacterial prostatitis: fluoroquinolone or TMP-SMX for 4–6 weeks; consider α-blocker adjunct for LUTS; recurrent cases need urology input.

5. Chronic pelvic pain syndrome (CP/CPPS): multimodal — education, pelvic-floor physio, α-blocker trial, NSAIDs, neuropathic pain agents (amitriptyline/gabapentin), CBT; avoid prolonged empiric antibiotics without evidence of infection.

C. PROSTATE CANCER (PRIMARY-CARE SCOPE)

1. Screening: Shared decision for men 55–69 y (USPSTF grade C); consider earlier (age 45–55) in higher-risk groups (Black men, strong FHx, BRCA1/2). Not routinely for ≥70 y or limited life expectancy.

2. Discuss benefits/harms (overdiagnosis, biopsy risks). If screening chosen: PSA with/without DRE at intervals (e.g., q2–4 y if low PSA). Abnormal PSA/DRE → urology for MRI-based risk assessment/biopsy.

3. Active surveillance is common for low-risk disease; definitive therapy (surgery/radiation) for higher-risk — oncology/urology-led. Manage treatment adverse effects (ED, incontinence, bowel symptoms) in collaboration.

DISPOSITION (DISCHARGE/OBSERVE/ TRANSFER) & RETURN PRECAUTIONS

1. Immediate ED/transfer: septic patient with suspected ABP (fever, rigors, hypotension), acute urinary retention with severe pain/renal failure, suspected cauda equina (urinary retention + saddle anesthesia/ leg weakness), gross hematuria with clots/obstruction.

2. Urgent (days) urology: recurrent retention, rising creatinine/hydronephrosis, persistent gross hematuria, abnormal DRE or significantly elevated/ repeat-elevated PSA, failure of medical therapy for LUTS, recurrent febrile UTIs.

3. Return immediately for: fever/chills, worsening pain, inability to pass urine, flank pain, new neurologic deficits, or new bone pain/weight loss.

PEARLS & PITFALLS

1. Don't check PSA during acute prostatitis/UTI/retention; repeat after recovery (6–8+ weeks).

2. 5-ARIs halve PSA — remember to adjust interpretation after ≥6 months of therapy.

3. In ABP, avoid vigorous DRE/massage and avoid urethral instrumentation when possible (risk of bacteremia).

4. Before adding antimuscarinics for storage LUTS, ensure low PVR to reduce retention risk.

5. Review medications that worsen retention (anticholinergics/α-agonists/opioids) and deprescribe

when possible.

REFERENCES

1. NICE CKS. Lower urinary tract symptoms in men; Urinary retention; Prostatitis (acute and chronic); Suspected cancer: recognition and referral — prostate (public). cks.nice.org.uk / nice.org.uk

2. AUA (American Urological Association) — Public guideline summaries: BPH/LUTS, Acute Urinary Retention, Prostatitis, Early Detection of Prostate Cancer (public summaries). auanet.org

3. EAU (European Association of Urology) — Guidelines (open PDFs) on Male LUTS, Prostate Cancer, Urological Infections (epididymo-orchitis/prostatitis). uroweb.org

4. AAFP. Acute Bacterial Prostatitis; Chronic Prostatitis/ Chronic Pelvic Pain Syndrome; Urinary Retention in Adults; BPH: Diagnosis and Management; Prostate Cancer Screening (open). aafp.org

5. USPSTF. Prostate Cancer Screening Recommendation Statement (2018, update in progress — public). uspreventiveservicestaskforce.org

6. CDC. STI Treatment Guidelines (urethritis/epididymitis) relevant to STI-associated prostatitis. cdc.gov

TESTICULAR PAIN — TORSION VS EPIDIDYMITIS (OFFICE/URGENT CARE)

OVERVIEW & "DON'T MISS"

1. Acute scrotal pain requires rapid exclusion of testicular torsion — a time-critical surgical emergency. Salvage chances are highest within ~6 hours and fall sharply thereafter.

2. Common etiologies: testicular torsion; torsion of testicular appendage; epididymitis/epididymo-orchitis (STI-related in younger, enteric in older); trauma; inguinal hernia/strangulation; renal colic; referred pain.

3. DON'T MISS: testicular torsion (sudden severe unilateral pain ± nausea/vomiting, high-riding horizontal testis, absent cremasteric reflex), incarcerated hernia, Fournier's gangrene, mumps orchitis (post-pubertal), tumor presenting with pain after torsion/infarct.

HISTORY & EXAM

1. Onset: sudden (torsion) vs gradual (epididymitis). Associated: nausea/vomiting (torsion), fever/dysuria/

urethral discharge (epididymitis).

2. Sexual/urinary history: new partners, insertive anal sex (enteric coverage), STI exposure, recent UTI, instrumentation/trauma, strenuous activity.

3. Exam: inspect position/lie (high-riding, transverse = torsion), scrotal edema/erythema, epididymal tenderness (posterolateral), cord thickening. Check cremasteric reflex (often absent in torsion). 'Prehn sign' is unreliable. Examine abdomen/inguinal region for hernia; check for costovertebral angle tenderness.

4. Peds: epididymitis is uncommon pre-puberty — consider anatomic anomalies/UTI; torsion of appendix testis shows 'blue-dot' sign.

DIFFERENTIAL DIAGNOSIS (TOP 5)

1. Testicular torsion.

2. Epididymitis/epididymo-orchitis (STI vs enteric).

3. Torsion of testicular/epididymal appendage.

4. Incarcerated/strangulated inguinal hernia.

5. Trauma/hematoma; less often: renal colic, tumor, varicocele, idiopathic scrotal edema (kids).

INVESTIGATIONS (POC/LABS/IMAGING)

1. High suspicion of torsion → do NOT delay urologic consultation/exploration for imaging.

2. If suspicion is low–moderate and access is rapid: color Doppler ultrasound (absent or decreased intratesticular flow suggests torsion; increased

epididymal flow/enlargement suggests epididymitis).

3. Urinalysis ± urine culture; NAAT for Chlamydia trachomatis/Neisseria gonorrhoeae when STI risk; consider CRP/WBC if systemic features (non-specific).

4. Consider scrotal POCUS if skilled, but negative POCUS does not rule out torsion if clinical concern persists.

MANAGEMENT (NON-PHARM → MEDS → PROCEDURES)

A. NON-PHARMACOLOGIC

1. Analgesia (acetaminophen/NSAIDs unless contraindicated). Scrotal elevation/support and ice for epididymitis. Rest and avoid strenuous activity/sexual intercourse until resolution.

2. Vaccinate for mumps if non-immune (prevention of orchitis).

B. MEDICATIONS (EXAMPLES; VERIFY LOCAL GUIDANCE & CONTRAINDICATIONS)

1. Epididymitis likely due to chlamydia/gonorrhea (typical age <35, new partner, no insertive anal sex):

2. Ceftriaxone 500 mg IM once (1 g if ≥150 kg) + doxycycline 100 mg PO BID × 10 days.

3. Epididymitis in men who practice insertive anal sex (cover STI + enteric):

4. Ceftriaxone 500 mg IM once (1 g if ≥150 kg) +

levofloxacin 500 mg PO daily × 10 days.

5.   Epididymitis due to enteric organisms only (older men, urinary tract pathology, post-instrumentation; low STI risk):

6.   Levofloxacin 500 mg PO daily × 10 days (or ofloxacin 300 mg PO BID × 10 days where used).

7.   Adjuncts: consider doxycycline alternatives if intolerance (e.g., azithromycin 1 g once then 500 mg daily × 2–4 days per local protocol, though evidence is weaker). Treat sexual partners per STI protocols; abstain until 7 days after both finish therapy and symptoms resolve.

C. PROCEDURES

1.   Suspected torsion: immediate urologic consultation for surgical exploration and bilateral orchiopexy. Do not delay for imaging if high suspicion.

2.   If immediate OR unavailable and high suspicion: attempt gentle manual detorsion as a bridge — usually 'open-book' rotation (lateral) of the affected testis 180–360°; pain relief and lowering of testis suggest success. Confirm with Doppler as soon as possible and still proceed to orchiopexy.

3.   Torsion of testicular appendage: supportive care (NSAIDs, rest, scrotal support); surgical excision if persistent severe pain or diagnostic uncertainty.

4.   Epididymitis: ensure follow-up in 48–72 h to confirm clinical improvement; evaluate for abscess if worsening.

DISPOSITION (DISCHARGE/OBSERVE/ TRANSFER) & RETURN PRECAUTIONS

1. Immediate ED/urology: high suspicion torsion (sudden severe unilateral pain, high-riding testis, absent cremasteric reflex, nausea/vomiting), suspected incarcerated hernia, scrotal necrotizing infection, testicular rupture after trauma, sepsis.

2. Outpatient: uncomplicated epididymitis responding to therapy; provide written precautions.

3. Return immediately for: increasing pain/swelling, fever/chills, vomiting, new urinary retention, inability to tolerate PO, or no improvement within 48–72 h.

PEARLS & PITFALLS

1. Torsion is a CLINICAL diagnosis — normal UA and even equivocal ultrasound do not exclude it when suspicion is high.

2. Cremasteric reflex absent strongly supports torsion, but presence does not fully exclude it.

3. 'Prehn sign' is unreliable — don't use to rule out torsion.

4. In prepubertal boys, epididymitis is uncommon; look for anatomic/UT causes and consider antibiotics targeting urinary pathogens.

5. Always screen and treat STIs for patients and partners when indicated; counsel abstinence until treatment is completed and symptoms resolve.

REFERENCES

1. CDC. 2021–2024 Sexually Transmitted Infections Treatment Guidelines — Epididymitis section (open). cdc.gov

2. AAFP. Testicular Torsion: Diagnosis, Evaluation, and Management; Epididymitis: An Overview (open articles). aafp.org

3. NICE CKS. Scrotal pain and swelling; Epididymo-orchitis (public). cks.nice.org.uk

4. Royal Children's Hospital (Melbourne). Acute scrotal pain guideline (open). rch.org.au

5. Emergency Care BC. Acute Scrotum; Testicular Torsion clinical summaries (public). emergencycarebc. ca

6. StatPearls (NCBI Bookshelf). Testicular Torsion; Epididymitis (open). ncbi.nlm.nih.gov/books

RESPIRATORY (ADULTS)

ASTHMA & COPD — FAMILY MEDICINE OFFICE

OVERVIEW & "DON'T MISS"

1. Asthma: variable respiratory symptoms (wheeze, SOB, chest tightness, cough) and variable expiratory airflow limitation.
2. COPD: persistent respiratory symptoms and airflow limitation due to airway/alveolar abnormalities from exposure (e.g., tobacco, biomass).
3. DON'T MISS (both): impending respiratory failure, status asthmaticus, severe COPD exacerbation with hypercapnic respiratory failure, pneumothorax, PE, ACS, pneumonia, anaphylaxis.

HISTORY & EXAM

1. Triggers/exposures: allergens, viral, exercise, cold air (asthma); tobacco/biomass/occupational (COPD). Nocturnal symptoms; SABA use frequency; exacerbations; hospitalizations/intubations.
2. Comorbidities: rhinitis/sinusitis, GERD, obesity/OSA, anxiety/depression, cardiac disease. Medication use/

adherence and inhaler technique.

3. Exam: vitals, SpO_2, accessory muscles, wheeze vs quiet chest, prolonged expiration; cyanosis/edema (cor pulmonale). Red flags: drowsiness, silent chest, speaking in words, PEF <50% predicted/best.

DIFFERENTIAL DIAGNOSIS (TOP 5)

1. Asthma vs COPD vs asthma–COPD overlap (ACO).
2. Upper airway: vocal cord dysfunction, laryngitis, foreign body (acute).
3. Cardiac: heart failure; ischemia causing dyspnea/ wheeze ('cardiac asthma').
4. Pulmonary: pneumonia, PE, pneumothorax/interstitial lung disease.
5. Other: deconditioning/obesity, GERD-related cough/ wheeze.

INVESTIGATIONS (POC/LABS/IMAGING)

1. Peak expiratory flow (PEF) at presentation and after bronchodilator; establish personal best for action plans.
2. Spirometry (stable):
3. Asthma: variable airflow limitation — FEV_1 increase ≥12% and ≥200 mL post-bronchodilator; excessive PEF variability (>10%).
4. COPD: post-BD FEV_1/FVC <0.70 confirms persistent airflow limitation (interpret with age).
5. CXR during exacerbations if fever, chest pain, focal

signs, or atypical course. ABG/VBG in severe cases (suspected hypercapnia).

6. Labs as indicated: CBC (eosinophils), BMP; viral testing when it changes management. Consider α-1 antitrypsin level if early-onset, minimal smoking, or family history.

MANAGEMENT (NON-PHARM → MEDS → PROCEDURES)

A. NON-PHARMACOLOGIC (BOTH)

1. Smoking cessation (behavioral + pharmacotherapy), vaccinations (influenza, COVID-19, pneumococcal, Tdap), inhaler technique check every visit, written action plan, trigger avoidance (asthma), pulmonary rehabilitation (COPD).

2. Oxygen: target 92–96% (asthma) and 88–92% (COPD exacerbation) pending ABG.

B. MEDICATIONS — CHRONIC CONTROL

1. ASTHMA (track aligned with modern GINA principles):

2. Reliever preferred: low-dose ICS-formoterol as needed across steps; alternative: SABA taken with concomitant ICS each time for mild disease.

3. Step-up (persistent symptoms/exacerbations): maintain ICS-formoterol (maintenance-and-reliever therapy) at low → medium dose; add LAMA if uncontrolled; evaluate for biologics (anti-IgE/IL-5/ IL-4Rα) at severe step.

4. Never use LABA without ICS in asthma.

5. COPD (aligned with GOLD A/B/E):

6. Group A: any bronchodilator (SABA/SAMA PRN or LABA/LAMA).

7. Group B (dyspnea): start LABA+LAMA dual bronchodilator.

8. Group E (exacerbation-prone): LABA+LAMA; add ICS if blood eosinophils high (≥300 cells/μL, or ≥100 with frequent exacerbations).

9. ICS risks: ↑ pneumonia risk; favor in eosinophilic phenotype/frequent exacerbations; avoid ICS monotherapy.

10. Consider roflumilast (chronic bronchitis, FEV_1 <50% with frequent exacerbations) or chronic macrolide (selected non-smokers with frequent exacerbations) under specialist guidance.

C. MEDICATIONS — ACUTE EXACERBATIONS (OFFICE/URGENT CARE)

1. ASTHMA:

2. Short-acting bronchodilator: SABA via MDI + spacer (4–8 puffs q20 min × 1 h) or neb; or use ICS-formoterol reliever if available per plan.

3. Systemic corticosteroid: prednisone 40–50 mg PO daily 5–7 days (children: 1–2 mg/kg/day, max 40–50 mg).

4. Adjuncts: ipratropium in moderate–severe; IV magnesium sulfate 2 g over 20 min for severe/

life-threatening; consider epinephrine for anaphylaxis. Observe response by PEF/SpO$_2$/clinical.

5. COPD:

6. Bronchodilators: SABA ± SAMA (albuterol ± ipratropium) via MDI/spacer or neb.

7. Systemic corticosteroid: prednisone 40 mg PO daily × 5 days.

8. Antibiotics if increased dyspnea, sputum volume AND/OR purulence, or need for ventilation: amoxicillin-clavulanate, doxycycline, or azithromycin depending on local resistance/allergy (5–7 days).

9. Consider NIV for acute hypercapnic respiratory failure; arrange ED transfer if needed.

DISPOSITION (DISCHARGE/OBSERVE/ TRANSFER) & RETURN PRECAUTIONS

1. Immediate ED/transfer: altered mental status, silent chest, cyanosis, SpO$_2$ <90% on air, PEF <50% best/ pred after initial treatment, rising PaCO$_2$, severe work of breathing, hemodynamic instability, suspected pneumothorax/PE/ACS.

2. Discharge when improved to mild symptoms with PEF ≥60–80% best/pred, stable SpO$_2$, and clear plan. Provide written action plan, inhaler technique review, and follow-up in 2–7 days (earlier if severe).

3. Return immediately for: worsening breathlessness, needing reliever more than q3–4 h, nighttime deterioration, confusion, chest pain, fever with purulent sputum.

PEARLS & PITFALLS

1. Check inhaler technique and adherence before stepping up therapy.
2. Consider AAT deficiency testing in COPD with onset <45, minimal smoking, or family history.
3. Overuse of SABA increases risk — ensure anti-inflammatory therapy in asthma (ICS).
4. ICS in COPD works best with higher eosinophils; reassess if recurrent pneumonias.
5. Step down asthma controller when controlled ≥3 months and risk low; keep some ICS on board.

REFERENCES

1. GINA — Global Initiative for Asthma. Global Strategy & Pocket Guide (public). ginasthma.org
2. GOLD — Global Initiative for Chronic Obstructive Lung Disease. Global Strategy & Pocket Guide (public). goldcopd.org
3. NICE CKS. Asthma; COPD; Acute exacerbations (public). cks.nice.org.uk
4. AAFP. Office Management of Asthma; COPD: Diagnosis and Management; Exacerbations (open articles). aafp.org
5. CDC. Asthma patient education & inhaler technique resources (public). cdc.gov
6. Canadian Thoracic Society & British Thoracic Society open summaries on asthma/COPD care and exacerbations (public). lung.ca / brit-thoracic.org.uk

RESPIRATORY INFECTIONS — URTI, SINUSITIS, BRONCHITIS, PNEUMONIA

OVERVIEW & "DON'T MISS"

1. URTI/acute cough are commonly viral (rhinovirus, influenza, RSV, SARS-CoV-2). Antibiotics rarely indicated except confirmed bacterial sinusitis or pneumonia.

2. Sinusitis: suspect bacterial only with (any): symptoms ≥10 days without improvement; severe onset with fever ≥39°C & purulent discharge/facial pain ≥3–4 days; or 'double-worsening' after initial improvement.

3. Acute bronchitis: cough ± sputum up to 3 weeks, often viral; rule out pneumonia (tachypnea, focal consolidation, hypoxia) and pertussis (paroxysms, inspiratory whoop, post-tussive emesis).

4. Community-acquired pneumonia (CAP): cough, fever, dyspnea, pleuritic pain + new infiltrate on chest X-ray. Assess severity (e.g., CURB-65, vitals, hypoxia).

5. DON'T MISS: severe sepsis/respiratory failure, epiglottitis, peritonsillar/retropharyngeal abscess, meningitis (URI→neck stiffness/AMS), influenza/RSV/

COVID-19 in high-risk, pulmonary embolism, TB (risk factors), necrotizing pneumonia, Lemierre syndrome (sore throat + neck pain/sepsis).

HISTORY & EXAM

1. Onset/duration, fever pattern, sick contacts/outbreaks, travel; vaccine status (flu/COVID-19, pertussis, pneumococcal).

2. Symptoms: rhinorrhea, sore throat, otalgia, facial pressure, purulent nasal discharge, cough (dry/productive), dyspnea, chest pain, hemoptysis, wheeze; red flags (confusion, dehydration, severe pleuritic pain).

3. Risk: COPD/asthma, CHF, diabetes, CKD, immunosuppression, pregnancy, age <2 or ≥65, smoking; aspiration risk (neuro, ETOH).

4. Exam: vitals incl. SpO_2; HEENT (tonsils, peritonsillar bulge, sinus tenderness, otitis media), lungs (rales/egophony/consolidation), heart, hydration; chest wall tenderness; calf tenderness if PE suspected.

DIFFERENTIAL DIAGNOSIS (TOP 5)

1. Viral URTI (common cold), influenza, COVID-19.

2. Acute bacterial rhinosinusitis.

3. Acute bronchitis (viral) vs pertussis.

4. Community-acquired pneumonia (typical/atypical).

5. Asthma/COPD exacerbation; less often: heart failure, PE.

INVESTIGATIONS (POC/LABS/IMAGING)

1. URTI/bronchitis: usually none. Consider rapid influenza/COVID-19 testing when results change management (antivirals/isolation).

2. Sinusitis: no imaging initially. CT sinuses only for suspected complications (orbital/intracranial) or recurrent/atypical.

3. Pneumonia suspected: chest X-ray to confirm; pulse oximetry. CBC ± BMP if moderate severity; consider CRP where available to support diagnosis; blood cultures not needed in outpatients unless severe.

4. Strep pharyngitis if indicated: Centor/McIsaac → RADT ± culture. Pertussis PCR in prolonged paroxysmal cough outbreaks/contacts.

5. Consider pregnancy test if doxycycline/fluoroquinolone contemplated in women of childbearing potential.

MANAGEMENT (NON-PHARM → MEDS → PROCEDURES)

A. NON-PHARMACOLOGIC (ALL)

1. Reassurance; fluids; rest; honey for cough (adults/ children >1 y); humidified air/saline irrigation for rhinitis/sinus symptoms; acetaminophen/NSAIDs for fever/myalgias (avoid NSAIDs if risk).

2. Educate about expected course: viral URTI 7–10 d; cough up to 3 wks (bronchitis). Safety-net and return precautions below.

3. Avoid routine antibiotics for URTI/bronchitis; avoid codeine in children and benzodiazepines/sedatives.

B. MEDICATIONS (EXAMPLES; VERIFY LOCAL RESISTANCE & CONTRAINDICATIONS)

1. Viral URTI: symptomatic only. Consider intranasal ipratropium for rhinorrhea; decongestants short-term in adults; avoid routine antibiotics/steroids.

2. Influenza (within 48 h or severe/high-risk): oseltamivir 75 mg BID × 5 d (dose adjust renal) or baloxavir (single dose) per eligibility.

3. Acute bacterial rhinosinusitis (adults):

4. First-line: amoxicillin-clavulanate 875/125 mg BID (or 500/125 mg TID) × 5–7 d.

5. Penicillin allergy (non-anaphylactic): doxycycline 100 mg BID × 5–7 d.

6. Severe β-lactam allergy: respiratory fluoroquinolone (e.g., levofloxacin) × 5 d — reserve for failures/intolerance.

7. Adjuncts: intranasal corticosteroid (e.g., mometasone) if allergic rhinitis; saline irrigation.

8. Acute bronchitis: NO antibiotics. Consider bronchodilator trial if wheeze/reactive airway. Pertussis: azithromycin 500 mg day 1 then 250 mg daily days 2–5 (or clarithromycin 500 mg BID × 7 d); prophylax close contacts per public health.

9. Community-acquired pneumonia (outpatient adults): treat minimum 5 d and clinically stable (afebrile 48–72

h, HR <100, RR <24, SpO$_2$ ≥90%).

10. No comorbidities: amoxicillin 1 g PO TID OR doxycycline 100 mg BID. Macrolide monotherapy only if local pneumococcal resistance <25%.

11. With comorbidities (chronic heart/lung/liver/ kidney disease; diabetes; alcoholism; malignancy; asplenia): amox-clav (high-dose) or cefuroxime/ cefpodoxime PLUS azithromycin/clarithromycin OR doxycycline; ALTERNATIVE monotherapy: respiratory fluoroquinolone (levofloxacin 750 mg daily or moxifloxacin 400 mg daily).

12. COPD exacerbation (if present): antibiotics only when increased dyspnea, sputum purulence, and volume (Anthonisen) or severe; 5 d typical (e.g., amox-clav, doxycycline, azithromycin).

C. PROCEDURES/REFERRALS

1. Nebulized bronchodilators for wheeze/reactive airway; spacer teaching.

2. ENT referral for recurrent sinusitis, nasal polyps, suspected complications; pulmonology for recurrent pneumonia, hemoptysis, or persistent abnormal CXR; infectious diseases for severe/atypical infections.

DISPOSITION (DISCHARGE/OBSERVE/ TRANSFER) & RETURN PRECAUTIONS

1. Immediate ED/transfer: SpO$_2$ <90% at rest, RR ≥30, hypotension, confusion, sepsis criteria,

severe dehydration, inability to tolerate PO, rapidly progressive swelling/pain of face/eye (orbital complications), drooling/stridor, severe chest pain or hemoptysis.

2. Outpatient: most URTIs/bronchitis and mild sinusitis/ CAP with reliable follow-up in 48–72 h.

3. Return immediately for: worsening dyspnea, persistent fever >72 h on therapy, confusion, severe facial pain/ swelling/visual changes, new chest pain, syncope.

PEARLS & PITFALLS

1. Use 'double-worsening/≥10-day' criteria to curb unnecessary sinusitis antibiotics.

2. No antibiotics for acute bronchitis; consider pertussis in prolonged cough outbreaks.

3. Always check local macrolide resistance before macrolide monotherapy for CAP; doxycycline or high-dose amoxicillin are reliable choices.

4. Assess oxygen saturation on room air; hypoxia is pneumonia until proven otherwise.

5. Vaccines prevent disease: annual influenza, COVID-19 boosters, pneumococcal (PCV20 or PCV15→PPSV23 when eligible), and Tdap (pertussis).

REFERENCES

1. IDSA/ATS. 2019 Community-Acquired Pneumonia in Adults Guideline (open access). thoracic.org / idsociety.org

2. NICE CKS. Acute sinusitis; Acute cough (including acute bronchitis); Pneumonia — community-acquired (public). cks.nice.org.uk

3. AAFP. Acute Rhinosinusitis in Adults; Acute Bronchitis; Community-Acquired Pneumonia: Outpatient Treatment (open articles). aafp.org

4. CDC. Antibiotic Stewardship — Outpatient; Influenza antiviral guidance; COVID-19 testing/isolation (public). cdc.gov

5. WHO. Clinical management of COVID-19 (public). who.int

6. Public Health Agency (national/provincial/state) advisories for influenza/RSV/COVID-19 seasons and pertussis outbreaks (public).

CO POISONING, SMOKE INHALATION & WILDFIRE AIR QUALITY

OVERVIEW & "DON'T MISS"

1. CO: colorless, odorless gas from combustion (heaters, vehicles, fires). Binds Hb with high affinity → tissue hypoxia; standard SpO_2 is unreliable.

2. Smoke inhalation: combination of thermal injury, particulates, irritant gases; may include CO and hydrogen cyanide (HCN).

3. Wildfire smoke: population-level exposure causing cardiorespiratory morbidity; counsel using AQHI levels and mitigation.

4. DON'T MISS: suspected CO exposure with headache, dizziness, syncope, confusion, chest pain, seizure; soot in nares/oropharynx, stridor, or signs of airway injury; lactate ≥10 mmol/L suggesting cyanide toxicity; pregnant patients (fetal risk).

HISTORY & EXAM

1. Exposure history: enclosed space heating, generators, garages, structure fire, time of exposure, others

symptomatic, CO alarm.

2. Symptoms: neurologic (HA, confusion, syncope), chest pain, dyspnea, N/V; for smoke: cough, wheeze, hoarseness, soot, facial burns.

3. Medical: CAD, COPD/asthma, pregnancy, anemia; meds/substances (smoking ↑ baseline COHb).

4. Exam: vitals; airway/voice/stridor; oropharyngeal/ nares soot; mental status; lungs; skin cherry hue is unreliable; pulse CO-ox if available.

DIFFERENTIAL DIAGNOSIS (TOP 5)

1. Influenza/viral illness causing headache & malaise after heater use (consider CO).

2. Migraine/vestibular disorders vs. CO-related headache/dizziness.

3. ACS/arrhythmia precipitated by hypoxia vs. primary cardiac disease.

4. Cyanide toxicity from smoke inhalation (high lactate, severe neurologic dysfunction).

5. Methemoglobinemia (oxidant exposure) causing hypoxia with normal PaO_2.

INVESTIGATIONS (POC/LABS/IMAGING)

1. COHb level via blood gas co-oximetry (preferred). Normals: nonsmokers ≤2–3%; smokers up to ~9%; symptomatic often ≥10%.

2. ABG/VBG with lactate; basic labs (CBC, BMP), troponin if chest pain/CAD risk; ECG.

3. CXR for smoke inhalation; consider CT if concern for airway injury/inhalation burns (specialist).

4. Pregnancy test in reproductive-potential patients; fetal monitoring if viable gestation.

5. Pulse oximetry is unreliable in CO; use multi-wavelength CO-oximetry if available.

MANAGEMENT (NON-PHARM → MEDS → PROCEDURES)

A. NON-PHARMACOLOGIC

1. Immediate removal from exposure; 100% oxygen by non-rebreather mask (or HFNC) until asymptomatic and COHb <5% (or <3% in pregnancy).

2. Airway management for smoke inhalation: early consideration of intubation if airway burns/stridor/voice change/edema.

3. Wildfire smoke: advise indoor clean air (close windows/doors when AQHI high, HEPA filtration/ portable air cleaner), reduce exertion, relocate to clean-air spaces if needed.

B. MEDICATIONS (EXAMPLES; INDIVIDUALIZE)

1. CO: 100% O_2 is primary therapy. Consider hyperbaric O_2 (HBO) with any of: COHb ≥25% (≥20% if pregnant), loss of consciousness, persistent neurologic deficits, severe acidosis (pH <7.1), end-organ ischemia (ischemic ECG/troponin), or pregnancy with COHb ≥15% (local protocols vary).

2. Cyanide (fire smoke): empiric hydroxocobalamin 5 g IV (may repeat once) when high suspicion (closed-space fire, soot + AMS, hypotension, lactate ≥10). Avoid nitrite-based kits in concurrent CO poisoning.

3. Bronchodilators for bronchospasm; inhaled corticosteroids or short oral burst for reactive airways per asthma/COPD plans during wildfire events.

4. Analgesia/antiemetics as needed.

C. PROCEDURES

1. Airway: early intubation if progressive edema; burn center consult as indicated.

2. Cardiac monitoring if chest pain/syncope/CAD; treat arrhythmias per ACLS (note CO can precipitate ischemia).

3. Public health: notify fire department/utility for CO source; advise CO detectors at home.

DISPOSITION (DISCHARGE/OBSERVE/ TRANSFER) & RETURN PRECAUTIONS

1. Discharge: asymptomatic, COHb normalized (<5% or local threshold), no pregnancy, normal exam/ ECG, safe environment; provide CO safety & smoke mitigation handout.

2. Observe/ED referral: persistent symptoms, elevated COHb, CAD/pregnancy, elevated troponin, smoke inhalation with respiratory symptoms, lactate elevation.

3. Transfer: HBO center for candidates; burn center for

airway burns/thermal injury; ICU if severe hypoxia, acidosis, or hemodynamic instability.

4. Return immediately for: recurrent headache, confusion, syncope, chest pain, dyspnea, or if home CO alarm sounds again.

PEARLS & PITFALLS

1. Standard SpO_2 can appear normal in CO poisoning — do not rely on it; use CO-oximetry.

2. Pregnancy is high-risk: treat aggressively and consider HBO at lower thresholds.

3. Lactate ≥10 mmol/L in a fire victim strongly suggests cyanide toxicity — give hydroxocobalamin promptly.

4. Asthma/COPD patients often need temporary step-up therapy during wildfire smoke; ensure action plans and inhaler access.

5. Prevention: install CO detectors on every floor; annual furnace inspection; never run engines indoors; create a clean-air room with HEPA during smoke events.

REFERENCES

1. CDC. Clinical Guidance for Carbon Monoxide (CO) Poisoning. Public: cdc.gov

2. NIOSH (CDC). Carbon Monoxide Hazards & Emergency Response; Wildfire Smoke & Worker Safety. Public: cdc.gov/niosh

3. Government of Canada / Health Canada. Carbon monoxide — risks and prevention; Wildfire smoke and

your health; Air Quality Health Index (AQHI). Public: canada.ca

4. BC Centre for Disease Control. Wildfire Smoke resources for clinicians and the public (open). Public: bccdc.ca

5. Emergency Care BC. Carbon Monoxide Poisoning — Clinical Summary (public). Public: emergencycarebc. ca

6. WHO. Carbon monoxide fact sheet; indoor air quality and household fuel safety (open). Public: who.int

7. U.S. EPA. Wildfire Smoke: A Guide for Public Health Officials (open). Public: epa.gov

GASTROENTEROLOGY
(ADULTS)

COMMON GASTROINTESTINAL DISEASES — FAMILY MEDICINE OFFICE

OVERVIEW & "DON'T MISS"

1. Frequent primary-care GI syndromes: GERD/ dyspepsia (± Helicobacter pylori), IBS vs IBD, acute diarrhea (incl. C. difficile), constipation, biliary colic/ cholecystitis, and MASLD/NAFLD.

2. DON'T MISS: GI bleeding (hematemesis/melena/ hematochezia), bowel obstruction/peritonitis, appendicitis, pancreatitis, cholangitis (fever + jaundice + RUQ pain), mesenteric ischemia (pain out of proportion), severe dehydration/electrolyte derangements, and new dysphagia/odynophagia or unintentional weight loss.

HISTORY & EXAM

1. Symptom pattern: onset/duration, relation to meals, nocturnal symptoms, alarm features (dysphagia, GI bleed, weight loss, anemia, persistent vomiting), bowel habit pattern per Bristol chart, stool blood/

mucus, fever, travel/food exposures, antibiotics (last 3 months), NSAIDs/alcohol.

2. Past/family hx: IBD, celiac, colorectal cancer/polyps; gallstones; liver disease; surgeries; pregnancy status.

3. Exam: vitals/orthostatics; hydration; focused oropharynx; abdomen (tenderness, guarding/rigidity, Murphy/McBurney, hepatosplenomegaly, masses); rectal exam if lower GI bleeding or obstruction suspected; skin for jaundice/spider angiomata; pelvic exam if indicated.

DIFFERENTIAL DIAGNOSIS (TOP 5)

1. GERD/dyspepsia (incl. H. pylori).
2. IBS (Rome IV) vs IBD (Crohn/UC).
3. Acute infectious diarrhea (viral/bacterial) including traveler's; C. difficile after antibiotics/health-care exposure.
4. Constipation (primary, medication-induced incl. opioids/anticholinergics, secondary metabolic).
5. Biliary colic/cholecystitis; consider MASLD/NAFLD in metabolic risk with elevated ALT.

INVESTIGATIONS (POC/LABS/IMAGING)

1. General screening (tailor): CBC (anemia), ferritin/iron studies (IDA), BMP (electrolytes/renal), ALT/AST/ALP/ bilirubin (cholestatic vs hepatocellular pattern).
2. Dyspepsia/GERD (<60 y, no alarms): 'test-and-treat' H. pylori (stool antigen or urea breath test). If ≥60 y or

alarm features → endoscopy.

3. H. pylori test of cure: 4+ weeks after antibiotics and 2+ weeks off PPIs (H2 blockers allowed) using UBT or stool antigen.

4. Chronic diarrhea: celiac serology (tTG-IgA + total IgA); fecal calprotectin or CRP to distinguish IBS from IBD when uncertainty; stool O&P/culture/antigen only if severe/prolonged, blood/fever, immunocompromised, travel, or outbreak.

5. Suspected C. difficile: stool NAAT or EIA per local algorithm only with diarrhea (≥3 unformed stools/day) and risk factors.

6. Constipation: usually clinical; consider TSH, calcium, glucose, meds review; avoid routine abdominal X-rays.

7. Biliary disease: RUQ ultrasound; lipase for suspected pancreatitis; cholestatic LFTs with jaundice warrant urgent evaluation.

8. MASLD/NAFLD: assess fibrosis risk with FIB-4 (age, AST, ALT, platelets) and consider elastography referral if indeterminate/high.

MANAGEMENT (NON-PHARM → MEDS → PROCEDURES)

A. NON-PHARMACOLOGIC

1. GERD/dyspepsia: weight reduction if overweight; avoid late meals (≥3 h before bed); elevate head of bed; limit alcohol, large/fatty meals, trigger foods; stop

NSAIDs when possible.

2. IBS: low-FODMAP trial (6–8 wks) then structured re-introduction; soluble fiber (psyllium); stress/sleep management; exercise; consider gut-directed CBT.

3. Diarrhea: oral rehydration solution (ORS); early re-feeding; hand hygiene; temporary lactose restriction if post-infectious.

4. Constipation: fluids as needed, regular physical activity, toileting routine; fiber (psyllium) with gradual titration.

5. MASLD: ≥7–10% weight loss target; Mediterranean-style diet; ≥150 min/wk activity (include resistance training); treat metabolic syndrome components (T2D, HTN, dyslipidemia); alcohol moderation/avoid heavy use.

B. MEDICATIONS (EXAMPLES; INDIVIDUALIZE & VERIFY LOCAL GUIDANCE)

1. GERD/dyspepsia: PPI once daily 30–60 min before breakfast for 4–8 wks; if response → step down to lowest effective dose/on-demand; if persistent → consider BID or EGD. H2RA for mild/infrequent symptoms.

2. H. pylori: 14-day bismuth quadruple therapy (PPI BID + bismuth subsalicylate/subcitrate QID + tetracycline QID + metronidazole TID/QID) where resistance unknown/high; confirm eradication (see above).

3. IBS-D: loperamide PRN; peppermint oil; bile-acid sequestrant if bile-acid diarrhea suspected; rifaximin

550 mg TID × 14 d (may repeat) where available; consider low-dose TCAs for pain (screen QT).

4. IBS-C: psyllium; polyethylene glycol; osmotic agents; consider secretagogues (linaclotide/plecanatide) or prucalopride where available if refractory.

5. Constipation (general): polyethylene glycol first-line; stimulant laxatives (senna/bisacodyl) PRN or short courses; docusate has limited benefit; treat OIC with osmotic + stimulant ± peripherally acting μ-opioid antagonists (e.g., naloxegol) if refractory.

6. Acute diarrhea: loperamide for non-bloody afebrile cases; avoid in dysentery/high fever. Traveler's diarrhea: azithromycin single dose (1 g) or short course per region; avoid fluoroquinolones in high resistance areas; no antibiotics for routine viral gastroenteritis.

7. C. difficile: oral fidaxomicin preferred or vancomycin per guideline; stop inciting antibiotics when possible; avoid anti-motility agents in severe disease; arrange follow-up.

8. Biliary colic: NSAIDs (e.g., ketorolac/ibuprofen) and surgical referral for symptomatic stones; suspected cholecystitis/cholangitis → ED.

9. MASLD: no routine pharmacotherapy in primary care unless specialist-directed; optimize diabetes meds (GLP-1 RA, SGLT2i) for weight/metabolic benefit where indicated.

C. PROCEDURES

1. Point-of-care urea breath test or stool antigen for H. pylori (before PPI/antibiotics as per protocols).

2. Anoscopy for suspected hemorrhoids/fissures if bleeding; fecal immunochemical test (FIT) for colorectal cancer screening per age/eligibility when asymptomatic.

3. Arrange endoscopy/colonoscopy via GI for alarm features, persistent symptoms, positive FIT, suspected IBD, iron-deficiency anemia, or recurrent GI bleeding.

DISPOSITION (DISCHARGE/OBSERVE/ TRANSFER) & RETURN PRECAUTIONS

1. Immediate ED/transfer: signs of shock or severe dehydration; peritonitis; GI bleeding with hemodynamic instability or ongoing hematemesis/melena; severe RUQ pain with fever/jaundice; suspected bowel obstruction or pancreatitis; intractable vomiting; severe dysphagia/food impaction.

2. Urgent GI/surgical referral (days): new-onset dysphagia, IDA, weight loss, persistent vomiting, abnormal LFTs (especially cholestatic), suspected IBD, recurrent biliary colic, persistent elevated FIB-4/ elastography concern.

3. Return immediately for: worsening pain, persistent fever, syncope, inability to keep fluids down, black/ bloody stools, or progressive jaundice/pruritus.

PEARLS & PITFALLS

1. Test for H. pylori in dyspepsia and peptic ulcer disease — and always confirm eradication.

2. Do not give antibiotics for most acute diarrhea; reserve for severe or specific indications.

3. Long-term PPI only when clearly indicated (severe erosive esophagitis, Barrett's, chronic NSAID users at high risk); reassess need periodically.

4. IBS is a positive diagnosis using Rome IV once red flags are excluded — avoid endless testing.

5. Not all rectal bleeding is hemorrhoids in adults over 50 — consider FIT/colonoscopy based on risk and guidelines.

REFERENCES

1. NICE CKS. Dyspepsia and GERD; Gastroenteritis; Constipation; Irritable Bowel Syndrome; Gallstones; Non-alcoholic Fatty Liver Disease (public). cks.nice.org.uk

2. AAFP. Dyspepsia and H. pylori 'test-and-treat'; Diagnosis and Management of IBS; Acute Diarrhea in Adults; Constipation in Adults; Gallstone Disease; Evaluation of Abnormal LFTs (open articles). aafp.org

3. CDC. Traveler's Diarrhea; C. difficile infection — clinician resources; Foodborne illnesses (public). cdc.gov

4. AASLD. Practice Guidance on MASLD/NAFLD (open access summaries & guidance). aasld.org

5. IDSA. Clinical Practice Guidelines for Infectious Diarrhea (2017, open). idsociety.org

6. AGA/ACG public patient/clinician resources: GERD, IBS, IBD basics, H. pylori (public pages). gastro.org / gi.org

7. WHO. Oral Rehydration Solution (ORS) guidance and composition (public). who.int

ABDOMINAL PAIN (ADULT)

OVERVIEW & "DON'T MISS"

1. Very common; etiologies vary by location (RUQ, epigastric, RLQ, LLQ, diffuse) and time course (acute vs. chronic).

2. DON'T MISS (time-sensitive emergencies): ruptured/ expanding AAA (older age, back pain, hypotension), mesenteric ischemia (pain out of proportion, AF), perforated viscus (sudden severe pain, peritonitis, free air), ectopic pregnancy (any reproductive-potential with pain/bleeding), bowel obstruction with strangulation (vomiting, distension, peritonitis), biliary sepsis/ ascending cholangitis, acute pancreatitis with organ failure, DKA/HHS presenting as abdominal pain.

3. Analgesia does not obscure surgical diagnoses — treat pain early while evaluating.

HISTORY & EXAM

1. OPQRST + location/radiation (e.g., RUQ → GB; flank → renal; epigastric → PUD/pancreas/MI). Associated symptoms: N/V, fever, jaundice, GI bleed, bowel habit changes, dysuria/hematuria, chest pain/SOB.

2. Risk factors: age, vascular disease/AF, alcohol, gallstones, prior abdominal surgery/adhesions, NSAIDs, recent antibiotics (C. difficile), travel, exposures, STI risk.

3. Women/pregnancy capable: menstrual/OB hx; last menstrual period; contraception; pregnancy test for all uncertain.

4. Exam: vitals incl. orthostatics; general appearance; abdomen (guarding, rebound, masses, Murphy, Rovsing, McBurney, CVA tenderness); hernias; rectal exam PRN; pelvic exam if lower abd pain/vaginal symptoms; testicular exam if indicated.

DIFFERENTIAL DIAGNOSIS (TOP 5)

1. Appendicitis (RLQ; migratory pain, anorexia, fever).

2. Biliary colic/acute cholecystitis (RUQ pain ± fever, Murphy sign).

3. Renal colic/ureteric stone (flank → groin pain, hematuria).

4. Acute pancreatitis (epigastric pain radiating to back, ↑lipase).

5. Small bowel obstruction (colicky pain, vomiting, distension, prior surgery).

INVESTIGATIONS (POC/LABS/IMAGING)

1. POC: vitals, capillary glucose; urine dip; pregnancy test (urine/serum hCG) for all with child-bearing potential.

2. Labs (tailor to presentation): CBC, electrolytes, creatinine, LFTs/ALP/bilirubin, lipase, CRP, lactate (ischemia/sepsis), urinalysis ± culture; troponin/ECG if epigastric/atypical chest pain.

3. Imaging: RUQ ultrasound for biliary disease; pelvic ultrasound for gynecologic/ectopic concerns; CT abdomen/pelvis with IV contrast for undifferentiated or suspected obstruction/perforation; non-contrast low-dose CT for suspected renal colic when needed (US first in younger/low-risk).

4. Avoid unnecessary imaging in young/otherwise well with clear benign diagnoses; follow ACR Appropriateness Criteria.

MANAGEMENT (NON-PHARM → MEDS → PROCEDURES)

A. NON-PHARMACOLOGIC

1. ABC, IV access; NPO initially if surgical pathology possible; isotonic IV fluids for dehydration/sepsis.

2. Early analgesia (e.g., IV acetaminophen, opioids titrated to effect); antiemetics (ondansetron, metoclopramide).

3. Bowel rest; consider oral rehydration if mild and stable; early mobilization when appropriate.

B. MEDICATIONS (EXAMPLES; INDIVIDUALIZE)

1. PPI for suspected peptic disease/upper GI bleed (e.g., pantoprazole).

2.   Antispasmodics/anticholinergics PRN for biliary/colicky pain (use judiciously).

3.   Antibiotics when indicated: suspected cholangitis/ cholecystitis, appendicitis, complicated diverticulitis, perforation, or sepsis (choose per local patterns; e.g., ceftriaxone + metronidazole, or piperacillin-tazobactam if severe).

4.   Glycemic control for DKA/HHS per protocol; treat precipitating causes.

5.   Avoid NSAIDs in suspected GI bleed, renal failure, or peptic ulcer complications.

C. PROCEDURES

1.   POCUS (if available): FAST-abdomen, gallbladder, aorta, renal hydronephrosis, urinary retention.

2.   NG tube for persistent vomiting or bowel obstruction with severe distension; Foley catheter for strict I/O monitoring in unstable patients.

3.   Early surgical/gynecology/urology consult when red flags or imaging/labs suggest operative pathology.

DISPOSITION (DISCHARGE/OBSERVE/ TRANSFER) & RETURN PRECAUTIONS

1.   Discharge: pain controlled with oral meds, tolerating PO, normal vitals, no red flags, clear diagnosis or safe undifferentiated pathway with close follow-up; provide return precautions.

2.   Observe/Same-day reassessment: diagnostic

uncertainty, new labs pending, moderate dehydration, or social concerns.

3. Transfer/Admit: hemodynamic instability, peritonitis, sepsis, obstruction, perforation, mesenteric ischemia, suspected AAA, uncontrolled pain/vomiting, pregnancy-related emergencies.

4. Return immediately for: worsening pain, fever, persistent vomiting, GI bleeding, syncope, chest pain, inability to keep fluids down.

PEARLS & PITFALLS

1. Treat pain early; it does not mask the exam or delay diagnoses when used appropriately.

2. Always test for pregnancy in reproductive-potential patients with abdominal pain—even if tubal ligation history.

3. Use quadrant-based approach + time course; correlate with risk factors (e.g., gallstones, alcohol, prior surgery).

4. CT with IV contrast is preferred for undifferentiated acute abdomen; ultrasound first for RUQ and gynecologic pathology; minimize radiation in young patients.

5. Re-examination over time is valuable — evolving signs often clarify the diagnosis.

REFERENCES

1. American College of Radiology (ACR) Appropriateness

Criteria® — Acute Nonlocalized Abdominal Pain, Right Upper Quadrant Pain, Suspected Appendicitis. Public: acsearch.acr.org

2. American Academy of Family Physicians (AAFP). Evaluation of Acute Abdominal Pain in Adults; Acute Abdominal Pain in Children (open articles). aafp.org

3. Merck Manual Professional. Abdominal Pain — Evaluation and Differential Diagnosis; Acute Abdomen. merckmanuals.com

4. NICE Clinical Knowledge Summaries (CKS). Abdominal pain — acute (adult). cks.nice.org.uk

5. Emergency Care BC — clinical summaries on common abdominal conditions (e.g., biliary colic/cholecystitis, appendicitis, pancreatitis, bowel obstruction). emergencycarebc.ca

6. Government of Canada — Foodborne illness & gastroenteritis public resources; public health advisories. canada.ca

COMMON ABDOMINAL CONDITIONS, IBD, CELIAC, MALABSORPTION SYNDROMES, H. PYLORI & GERD

OVERVIEW & "DON'T MISS"

1. IBD (Crohn/UC): chronic relapsing immune-mediated GI inflammation; Crohn = transmural, skip lesions; UC = continuous mucosal colitis starting at rectum.

2. Celiac disease: immune-mediated enteropathy triggered by gluten (wheat/barley/rye) in genetically susceptible (HLA-DQ2/DQ8).

3. Malabsorption syndromes: include pancreatic exocrine insufficiency (PEI), small intestinal bacterial overgrowth (SIBO), bile-acid diarrhea, short bowel, giardiasis, postsurgical states.

4. H. pylori: common cause of PUD, atrophic gastritis; test-and-treat strategy in dyspepsia/PUD; confirm eradication.

5. GERD: troublesome reflux symptoms ± esophagitis; diagnose clinically unless alarms (dysphagia, bleeding, weight loss).

6. DON'T MISS: toxic megacolon/fulminant colitis, severe GI bleed, bowel obstruction/perforation, cholangitis in IBD-PSC, celiac crisis (rare), severe dehydration/ electrolyte derangements, alarm symptoms (dysphagia/weight loss/IDA).

HISTORY & EXAM

1. Red flags: nocturnal diarrhea, blood/mucus, weight loss, fever, persistent vomiting, dysphagia/ odynophagia, anemia, family history CRC/IBD/celiac.

2. IBD: stool frequency/urgency/tenesmus, abdominal pain pattern, perianal disease (fistula), extra-intestinal (uveitis, PSC, erythema nodosum, arthritis).

3. Celiac/malabsorption: chronic diarrhea/steatorrhea, bloating, iron-deficiency anemia, neuropathy, dermatitis herpetiformis, fractures, infertility; dietary gluten exposure.

4. H. pylori/dyspepsia: epigastric pain, NSAID use, prior PUD, bleeding history.

5. GERD: heartburn/regurgitation (post-prandial/ nocturnal), cough/hoarseness; triggers (late meals, caffeine, alcohol).

6. Exam: vitals/orthostatics; abdominal tenderness/ masses; perianal exam (Crohn); weight/BMI; signs of micronutrient deficiency; stool guaiac if indicated.

DIFFERENTIAL DIAGNOSIS (TOP 5)

1. IBS (functional) vs IBD (organic).

2. Infectious colitis (C. difficile, Campylobacter, Salmonella, Shigella, EHEC), parasites (Giardia).

3. Celiac vs non-celiac gluten sensitivity vs wheat allergy.

4. Peptic ulcer disease, functional dyspepsia, gastritis (H. pylori/NSAID).

5. PEI, SIBO, bile-acid diarrhea, hyperthyroidism/ diabetes-related gastroparesis.

INVESTIGATIONS (POC/LABS/IMAGING)

1. General: CBC (IDA, leukocytosis), ferritin/iron studies, B12/folate, CMP/LFTs, CRP/ESR; celiac serology where indicated; pregnancy test if applicable.

2. IBD suspected: fecal calprotectin to distinguish IBD from IBS (elevated in IBD); stool cultures incl. C. difficile in flares; colonoscopy with biopsies is diagnostic ± ileoscopy; imaging (CT/MR enterography) for small bowel or complications.

3. Celiac suspected: tissue transglutaminase IgA (tTG-IgA) + total IgA (to exclude deficiency). If IgA deficient → tTG-IgG or DGP-IgG. Positive serology → confirm with duodenal biopsies while ON gluten. HLA-DQ2/DQ8 negative makes celiac very unlikely.

4. Malabsorption work-up (tailored): fecal elastase (PEI), 72-h fecal fat or Sudan stain for steatorrhea, breath tests (glucose/lactulose) for SIBO, stool Giardia antigen, bile-acid diarrhea tests where available (or empirical bile-acid sequestrant trial).

5. H. pylori: stool antigen or urea breath test for initial dx; endoscopic biopsy if alarm features/ulcer complications. Test OF CURE at ≥4 weeks after therapy and ≥2 weeks off PPIs (H2 blockers OK).

6. GERD/dyspepsia: empiric PPI trial if <60 and no alarms; EGD if ≥60 or alarm features; consider H. pylori testing in dyspepsia ('test-and-treat').

MANAGEMENT (NON-PHARM → MEDS → PROCEDURES)

A. NON-PHARMACOLOGIC

1. IBD: smoking cessation (especially Crohn), vaccinations (influenza/COVID-19/pneumococcal/shingles), nutrition optimization (consider low-residue during flares), screen bone health; stress/sleep support; avoid NSAIDs when possible.

2. Celiac: strict, lifelong gluten-free diet with dietitian support; correct deficiencies (iron, folate, B12, vitamin D, calcium); vaccinate for hyposplenism considerations if present.

3. Malabsorption: tailored diet (e.g., low-fat with pancreatic enzyme therapy for PEI), rehydration, vitamin/mineral repletion.

4. H. pylori/GERD: lifestyle — avoid late meals (≥3 h), weight loss if overweight, elevate head of bed, limit alcohol/caffeine, stop smoking; avoid NSAIDs if PUD.

B. MEDICATIONS (EXAMPLES; VERIFY LOCAL GUIDANCE/RESISTANCE & CONTRAINDICATIONS)

1. IBD (primary-care scope): mild UC — 5-ASA (oral ± rectal); mild ileocecal Crohn — budesonide MMX/ CR. Systemic corticosteroids for moderate–severe flares are bridge therapy; maintenance and biologics/ immunomodulators are specialist-directed. Screen for C. difficile during flares.

2. Celiac: no role for steroids/biologics unless refractory celiac (specialist). Avoid gluten until after diagnostic testing is complete.

3. PEI: pancreatic enzyme replacement (e.g., pancrelipase with meals); fat-soluble vitamin supplementation; treat cause (chronic pancreatitis).

4. SIBO: treat underlying cause; short course antibiotics (e.g., rifaximin) per local protocols; caution with recurrence.

5. Bile-acid diarrhea: bile-acid sequestrants (cholestyramine/colesevelam) empiric trial where testing unavailable.

6. H. pylori (first-line where resistance unknown/high): 14-day bismuth quadruple therapy — PPI BID + bismuth subsalicylate/subcitrate QID + tetracycline QID + metronidazole TID/QID. Confirm eradication (see above).

7. GERD: PPI once daily 30–60 min before breakfast for 4–8 wks; if response → step down to lowest effective/ on-demand; partial response → consider BID or switch PPI. H2RA for mild/infrequent. Add alginate after meals PRN.

C. PROCEDURES

1. Arrange colonoscopy with biopsies for confirmed/ suspected IBD; EGD for alarm features/dysphagia/ IDA/PUD; MR/CT enterography for small bowel Crohn or complications.

2. Nutrition and bone density assessments in IBD/celiac; vaccinations before immunosuppression.

3. FIT/CRC screening per age/IBD risk protocols; PSC surveillance (with GI) when applicable.

DISPOSITION (DISCHARGE/OBSERVE/ TRANSFER) & RETURN PRECAUTIONS

1. Immediate ED/transfer: severe dehydration/shock, high fever with severe abdominal pain, peritonitis, suspected toxic megacolon (abdominal distension, systemic toxicity), GI bleed with instability, obstruction, severe dysphagia/food impaction.

2. Urgent GI (days): new IBD with significant symptoms, persistent IDA or weight loss, positive celiac serology needing biopsy, refractory GERD on optimized PPI, recurrent peptic ulcer, positive H. pylori test not responding to first-line therapy.

3. Return immediately for: worsening pain/fever, persistent bleeding, inability to keep fluids down, progressive dysphagia, syncope.

PEARLS & PITFALLS

1. Test for celiac BEFORE starting gluten-free diet; otherwise serology/biopsy may normalize.

2. Use fecal calprotectin to differentiate IBS from IBD and to monitor IBD activity alongside symptoms.

3. Always confirm H. pylori eradication — and ensure PPI hold (≥2 weeks) before test of cure.

4. Do not leave patients on long-term high-dose PPIs without indication — reassess and step down when possible.

5. Crohn smokers flare more — smoking cessation is a key 'medication'.

REFERENCES

1. NICE CKS. Inflammatory bowel disease; Coeliac disease; Dyspepsia and GERD; Diarrhoea; Irritable bowel syndrome (public). cks.nice.org.uk

2. AAFP. Inflammatory Bowel Disease: Diagnosis and Management; Celiac Disease: Common and Overlooked; Dyspepsia and H. pylori Test-and-Treat; Management of GERD (open articles). aafp.org

3. AGA/ACG public resources: IBD, Celiac, GERD, H. pylori (patient/clinician pages). gastro.org / gi.org

4. ECCO & Coeliac UK patient/professional resources

(open). ecco-ibd.eu / coeliac.org.uk

5. CDC. Traveler's Diarrhea; C. difficile; Giardia —
   clinician resources (public). cdc.gov

6. WHO. Oral Rehydration Solution (ORS) guidance
   (public). who.int

RECTAL BLEEDING (BRBPR / LOWER GI)

OVERVIEW & "DON'T MISS"

1. Rectal bleeding ranges from minor bright-red blood on tissue to large-volume hematochezia. Most outpatient cases are benign anorectal (hemorrhoids, fissures), but malignancy/colitis/diverticular or even brisk upper GI bleeding can present with hematochezia.

2. DON'T MISS: hemodynamic instability/orthostasis, ongoing large-volume bleeding, maroon stools with clots, melena (upper GI source), severe abdominal pain/fever (ischemic or infectious colitis), anemia symptoms (syncope, chest pain), anticoagulant/antiplatelet-associated bleeding, post-polypectomy bleed.

HISTORY & EXAM

1. Characterize bleeding: color (bright red vs maroon vs black), amount (streaks vs coating stool vs bowl full), frequency, mixed with stool or dripping, relation to defecation/straining, pain with BM (fissure), mucus/diarrhea (colitis).

2. Associated symptoms: abdominal pain/cramps, fever,

weight loss, change in bowel habits, constipation, tenesmus, dizziness/syncope; anal pruritus/lumps; recent procedures (colonoscopy/polypectomy).

3. Risk factors: age ≥40–50, family history of colorectal cancer/IBD, radiation, vascular disease (ischemia), infectious exposures, recent antibiotics (C. difficile), pregnancy/post-partum.

4. Medications: anticoagulants/antiplatelets, NSAIDs, iron/bismuth (black stools), constipation meds.

5. Exam: vitals incl. orthostatics; abdominal exam; external anal inspection; digital rectal exam (DRE) with anoscopy if available; stool color; look for fissure/hemorrhoids/masses; consider pelvic exam in women with unclear source.

DIFFERENTIAL DIAGNOSIS (TOP 5)

1. Hemorrhoids (painless bright-red blood, on paper/toilet, pruritus).

2. Anal fissure (severe pain with BM; streaks on stool).

3. Diverticular hemorrhage (sudden, painless, large-volume hematochezia).

4. Colitis (infectious, ischemic, inflammatory/IBD) — blood + diarrhea/abdominal pain/fever.

5. Colorectal neoplasia (polyps/cancer) — change in habits, iron-deficiency anemia, weight loss.

INVESTIGATIONS (POC/LABS/IMAGING)

1. Stable, low-risk minor BRBPR with obvious anorectal

source may not need labs; otherwise: CBC (Hb, MCV), ferritin/iron studies for chronic/occult loss, BMP (BUN/Cr), coagulation (INR) if on anticoagulants/bleeding, type & screen if moderate/heavy bleeding.

2. Stool tests: infectious stool PCR/culture/C. difficile if diarrhea/fever. Fecal occult blood/FIT are screening tools — not for acute visible bleeding.

3. Pregnancy test in women of reproductive age if imaging/meds could affect pregnancy.

4. Imaging/endoscopy: urgent ED pathway for hemodynamic instability or ongoing large bleed (resuscitation → CT angiography/endoscopic therapy). Outpatient colonoscopy for persistent/recurrent bleeding, age ≥40–50 without clear anorectal source, iron-deficiency anemia, or red-flag symptoms. Flexible sigmoidoscopy is an option in young low-risk with distal symptoms.

MANAGEMENT (NON-PHARM → MEDS → PROCEDURES)

A. NON-PHARMACOLOGIC (FOR MOST BENIGN ANORECTAL CAUSES)

1. Address constipation/straining: fiber 25–35 g/day (psyllium), fluids, stool softeners (PEG), avoid prolonged sitting on toilet; gentle perianal hygiene; sitz baths 10–15 min TID PRN.

2. Stop/limit NSAIDs; review anticoagulants/antiplatelets with risk–benefit (don't stop secondary-prevention

agents without plan).

3. Education: track amount/frequency; red-flag return precautions; keep iron-rich diet if anemic.

B. MEDICATIONS (EXAMPLES; VERIFY CONTRAINDICATIONS)

1. Hemorrhoids (symptomatic): topical hydrocortisone 1% cream/foam short course (≤7 days), topical anesthetics (lidocaine), witch-hazel pads; stool regulation and sitz baths are key.

2. Anal fissure: topical nitroglycerin 0.2–0.4% ointment pea-sized to anal canal BID–TID × 6–8 wks (warn headache/hypotension; avoid with PDE-5 inhibitors) OR topical calcium-channel blocker (diltiazem 2% or nifedipine 0.2–0.3% ointment) applied BID–TID. Consider topical lidocaine for pain.

3. Infectious colitis: treat organism (e.g., stop inciting antibiotics if C. difficile and follow local guideline). Avoid antimotility agents in dysentery/fever.

4. IBD flare: coordinate with GI; avoid NSAIDs; consider rectal mesalamine for distal UC if previously diagnosed.

5. Iron deficiency: oral elemental iron ~45–65 mg daily or every other day; consider IV iron for intolerance or severe depletion.

C. PROCEDURES/REFERRALS

1. ED transfer for ongoing brisk bleeding/instability (IV access, fluids, cross-match; GI/surgery).

2. Office procedures/Referrals: rubber-band ligation for grade II–III internal hemorrhoids; sclerotherapy/infrared coagulation as options. Chronic fissure refractory to meds → botulinum toxin injection or lateral internal sphincterotomy (colorectal surgery).

3. Outpatient colonoscopy for persistent/recurrent bleeding without clear anorectal source, iron-deficiency anemia, age ≥40–50, or red flags. Urgent CT angiography if active bleeding suspected and endoscopy not immediate.

DISPOSITION (DISCHARGE/OBSERVE/TRANSFER) & RETURN PRECAUTIONS

1. Immediate ED/transfer: SBP <100 mmHg, HR ≥100, orthostatic symptoms/syncope, ongoing large-volume bleeding or clots, maroon stools/melena, severe abdominal pain/fever, known cirrhosis/varices, anticoagulation with significant bleeding, post-polypectomy hemorrhage.

2. Outpatient management reasonable for: minor BRBPR with clear hemorrhoids/fissure, normal vitals, no anemia, reliable follow-up.

3. Return immediately for: increasing frequency/volume of blood, dizziness/weakness, black or maroon stools, persistent bleeding >48 h, new abdominal pain/fever.

PEARLS & PITFALLS

1. Not all 'hemorrhoids' — consider CRC, IBD, angiodysplasia, ischemic colitis, or brisk upper GI bleeding (especially with melena or elevated BUN:Cr).

2. Young patients with typical fissure/hemorrhoid and no red flags can be managed conservatively; persistent or atypical symptoms warrant endoscopic evaluation.

3. Resume indicated antithrombotics promptly after hemostasis; coordinate with cardiology for high-risk stents/AF.

4. Avoid rectal exam/manipulation in neutropenia or severe pain where fissure suspected — be gentle and defer if necessary.

5. Check ferritin for occult iron deficiency even if Hb normal in chronic low-grade bleeding.

REFERENCES

1. NICE CKS. Rectal bleeding — assessment and management (public). cks.nice.org.uk

2. AAFP. Acute Lower Gastrointestinal Bleeding: Evaluation and Management; Hemorrhoids: Diagnosis and Treatment; Anal Fissures: Diagnosis and Management (open articles). aafp.org

3. BSG (British Society of Gastroenterology) — Lower GI bleeding guidance (open summaries). bsg.org.uk

4. ACG/AGA patient & clinician public pages on lower GI bleeding and hemorrhoids/fissures (open summaries). gi.org / gastro.org

5. CDC. Colorectal Cancer — screening resources (public). cdc.gov
6. NICE NG12. Suspected cancer: recognition and referral — colorectal cancer (public). nice.org.uk

HEMATOLOGY & ONCOLOGY

ANEMIA (ADULT)

OVERVIEW & "DON'T MISS"

1. Anemia = low Hb/Hct for age/sex; classify by MCV (micro/normo/macro) and reticulocyte response (production vs. destruction/loss).

2. Common causes: iron deficiency (GI loss, menses), anemia of chronic disease/CKD, B12/folate deficiency, hemolysis, acute/chronic blood loss.

3. DON'T MISS: hemodynamic instability/active GI bleed; ACS precipitated by severe anemia; hemolysis with schistocytes (TTP/HUS/DIC), autoimmune hemolysis; new pancytopenia/leukemia; severe B12 deficiency with neurologic signs; pregnancy with severe anemia.

HISTORY & EXAM

1. History: fatigue, dyspnea, chest pain, palpitations, syncope; bleeding (melena/hematochezia, menorrhagia, epistaxis), pica; diet (iron/B12), alcohol; meds (NSAIDs, PPIs, methotrexate, hydroxyurea), chronic disease, CKD, thyroid/liver; family hx hemoglobinopathies; travel/exposures (lead).

2. Exam: vitals (orthostatics), pallor/jaundice,

glossitis/cheilitis, koilonychia, tachycardia/murmur, hepatosplenomegaly, lymphadenopathy, neurologic findings (paresthesias/ataxia), rectal exam if GI bleed suspected.

DIFFERENTIAL DIAGNOSIS (TOP 5)

1. Iron deficiency anemia (IDA) — GI blood loss until proven otherwise in men/post-menopausal women.
2. Anemia of chronic disease/inflammation ± CKD.
3. Vitamin B12 or folate deficiency (macrocytosis).
4. Hemolytic anemia (autoimmune, MAHA, G6PD, hereditary spherocytosis).
5. Mixed anemia (e.g., IDA + B12/folate) presenting with near-normal MCV.

INVESTIGATIONS (POC/LABS/IMAGING)

1. Initial labs: CBC with indices & smear, reticulocyte count, ferritin, serum iron/TIBC to calculate TSAT, B12, folate; creatinine/eGFR, TSH/LFTs as indicated; CRP if inflammation suspected.
2. Interpretation tips: ferritin <30 μg/L suggests IDA; with inflammation, consider IDA if ferritin <100 μg/L and TSAT <20%.
3. Hemolysis workup if suspected: LDH↑, indirect bilirubin↑, haptoglobin↓, reticulocytosis; direct antiglobulin test (DAT) for AIHA; smear for schistocytes/spherocytes.
4. Stool FIT/FOBT for occult blood if no overt GI

symptoms (not a substitute for endoscopy).

5. If IDA: evaluate source — premenopausal heavy menses vs. GI; men and post-menopausal women usually need bidirectional endoscopy; screen for celiac disease (tTG-IgA ± total IgA).

6. Consider pregnancy test in reproductive-potential patients; CKD workup if normocytic with low EPO context.

MANAGEMENT (NON-PHARM → MEDS → PROCEDURES)

A. NON-PHARMACOLOGIC

1. Dietary counselling: iron-rich foods (heme iron best), vitamin C with meals, avoid tea/coffee with iron; address menorrhagia (refer if needed).

2. Treat underlying cause: manage GI sources (ulcer, H. pylori), stop offending meds (e.g., NSAIDs when possible), manage chronic disease/CKD, alcohol reduction.

B. MEDICATIONS (EXAMPLES; INDIVIDUALIZE)

1. Oral iron for IDA: aim 40–65 mg ELEMENTAL iron once daily or every other day (better tolerance/ absorption than multiple daily dosing). Take on empty stomach or with vitamin C; separate from calcium/ PPIs. Expect Hb ↑ ~10 g/L (1 g/dL) every 2–3 weeks. Continue 3 months after Hb normal to replete stores.

2. IV iron for: oral intolerance/malabsorption, ongoing

blood loss, late pregnancy/severe anemia, CKD on ESA, need for rapid repletion. Choose formulation per availability; monitor for reactions.

3. Vitamin B12 deficiency: oral cyanocobalamin 1000 μg daily is effective in most; if severe neurologic symptoms, consider IM 1000 μg weekly × 4 then monthly. Recheck B12 and symptoms.

4. Folate deficiency: folic acid 1 mg daily (AFTER ruling out B12 deficiency to avoid masking neurologic injury).

5. Anemia of CKD: consider ESA per nephrology guidance after iron repletion; target Hb typically ≤115–120 g/L; avoid rapid rises.

6. Autoimmune hemolysis: urgent hematology input — steroids first-line; manage triggers and transfuse if needed.

C. PROCEDURES

1. Endoscopic evaluation for unexplained IDA (especially men/post-menopausal women) per GI referral pathways.

2. Transfusion: restrictive strategy for stable adults (consider at Hb <70 g/L, or <80 g/L with CVD or symptoms). Transfuse for instability/active bleeding regardless of Hb; coordinate with ED/hospital.

DISPOSITION (DISCHARGE/OBSERVE/ TRANSFER) & RETURN PRECAUTIONS

1. Discharge: stable, clear plan (iron/B12/folate), source

evaluation arranged, and follow-up labs in 2–4 weeks to confirm Hb response.

2. Observe/urgent review: symptomatic moderate anemia, uncertain source, or high risk for decompensation (elderly, CVD).

3. Transfer/ED: hemodynamic instability, active GI bleed, chest pain/ACS, syncope, Hb dangerously low, suspected TTP/HUS/DIC or severe hemolysis, pancytopenia, or pregnancy with severe anemia.

4. Return immediately for: melena/hematochezia, syncope, chest pain, dyspnea at rest, neurologic change.

PEARLS & PITFALLS

1. Always check reticulocyte count early — separates production failure from hemolysis/blood loss.

2. Ferritin is an acute-phase reactant — use TSAT and CRP when inflammation present.

3. Combined deficiencies can normalize MCV — look at RDW and smear.

4. Do not give folate before ruling out B12 deficiency.

5. In IDA, think 'why': GI cancer risk rises with age — don't skip source evaluation in men/post-menopausal women.

REFERENCES

1. NICE Clinical Knowledge Summaries (CKS). Anaemia — iron deficiency; Anaemia — B12 and folate

deficiency (public). cks.nice.org.uk

2. British Society for Haematology (BSH). Guidelines for the diagnosis and management of iron deficiency and B12/folate deficiency (open summaries). b-s-h.org.uk

3. American Academy of Family Physicians (AAFP). Evaluation of Anemia in Adults; Iron Deficiency Anemia: Evaluation and Management (open articles). aafp.org

4. World Health Organization (WHO). Haemoglobin concentrations for the diagnosis of anaemia and assessment of severity; WHO guidance on iron supplementation (public). who.int

5. BC Guidelines / Provincial pathways. Iron Deficiency — Diagnosis and Management; Anemia evaluation (public). bcguidelines.gov.bc.ca

6. Choosing Wisely Canada. Don't order unnecessary tests or transfusions in stable anemia (public). choosingwiselycanada.org

7. Merck Manual Professional. Anemia overview; Hemolytic anemia; Megaloblastic anemia (open). merckmanuals.com

LYMPHADENOPATHY — FAMILY MEDICINE

OVERVIEW & "DON'T MISS"

1. Definition: lymph node enlargement (>1 cm; epitrochlear >0.5 cm) — localized vs generalized (≥2 noncontiguous regions).

2. Most cases are benign/reactive (viral). Approach by age, duration, location, and red flags.

3. DON'T MISS: airway compromise (deep neck space infection), bacterial lymphadenitis/abscess, lymphoma/leukemia, metastatic head & neck or supraclavicular nodes (intra-abdominal/thoracic malignancy), TB/NTM, Kawasaki disease in children.

HISTORY & EXAM

1. Time course: acute (<2 wks), subacute (2–6 wks), chronic (>6 wks). Symptoms: fever, night sweats, weight loss, fatigue, pruritus, sore throat, dental pain, skin lesions, cat exposure/scratch, travel/TB exposure, sexual history, medications (phenytoin, allopurinol, hydralazine), vaccines.

2. Distribution: localized (drainage area exam: scalp/ ears/oral cavity, dental, skin) vs generalized (systemic causes).

3. Node features: size, tenderness, mobility, consistency (rubbery vs hard), matting, overlying skin; fixed, hard, non-tender nodes are more concerning.

4. Red flags: supraclavicular node, node >2 cm persisting >4–6 wks, generalized adenopathy, B-symptoms, abnormal bleeding/bruising, hepatosplenomegaly, abnormal chest exam/voice change, rapidly enlarging mass.

5. Children: look for signs of Kawasaki (≥5 days fever + mucocutaneous features) and deep neck infection (trismus, drooling, torticollis).

DIFFERENTIAL DIAGNOSIS (TOP 5)

1. Reactive viral (URTI, EBV/CMV, COVID-19) — tender, mobile, recent infection.

2. Acute bacterial lymphadenitis (Staph/Strep), dental/ skin source — tender, erythematous ± fluctuance.

3. Atypical infections: Bartonella henselae (cat scratch), TB/NTM, toxoplasmosis, syphilis, HIV.

4. Malignancy: lymphoma/leukemia; metastatic H&N/ thyroid/skin (esp. supraclavicular).

5. Autoimmune/inflammatory: SLE, sarcoidosis, serum sickness/drug reaction (DRESS).

INVESTIGATIONS (POC/LABS/IMAGING)

1. Targeted based on H&P; not every case needs labs on first visit.

2. Basic: CBC (anemia, leukocytosis/lymphocytosis), peripheral smear if blasts suspected; ESR/CRP; CMP; HIV (consent/risk), EBV/CMV serology if mono-like; TB testing (IGRA/TST) if risk; toxoplasma/syphilis serology when indicated.

3. Throat swab if pharyngitis; dental evaluation if oral/dental source suspected.

4. Ultrasound (first line in neck masses, esp. children): distinguishes solid vs cystic/abscess; malignant features — round shape, loss of fatty hilum, hypoechoic, necrosis, peripheral vascularity, matting.

5. CXR if persistent cervical/supraclavicular nodes or TB risk; CT/MRI for deep neck masses or if malignancy suspected (coordinate with ENT).

6. If malignancy strongly suspected or unexplained persistent nodes: tissue diagnosis. Prefer excisional biopsy for lymphoma; core needle acceptable in metastatic disease; FNA has limited sensitivity for lymphoma.

MANAGEMENT (NON-PHARM → MEDS → PROCEDURES)

A. NON-PHARMACOLOGIC

1. Observation: localized, small (<1–2 cm), soft, mobile

nodes after viral illness without red flags → watchful waiting with re-exam in 3–4 weeks.

2. Supportive care: analgesia, warm compresses for tender nodes; oral hygiene/dental care when relevant; wound care for nearby skin infections.

3. Counselling: avoid empiric steroids before diagnosis if malignancy suspected (can obscure pathology).

B. MEDICATIONS (EXAMPLES; INDIVIDUALIZE; CHECK LOCAL RESISTANCE/RENAL DOSING)

1. Acute unilateral bacterial cervical lymphadenitis (likely Staph/Strep; dental/skin source considered):

2. Adults: cephalexin 500 mg PO q6h or amoxicillin-clavulanate 875/125 mg PO BID × 5–7 d; add MRSA coverage if risk (e.g., doxycycline 100 mg BID or TMP-SMX) often combined with β-lactam for streptococcal coverage.

3. Children: cephalexin 25–50 mg/kg/day divided q6–8h OR amoxicillin-clavulanate 45 mg/kg/day divided BID; duration 5–7 d; reassess 48–72 h.

4. Cat scratch disease: azithromycin 500 mg day 1 then 250 mg daily days 2–5 (peds: 10 mg/kg day 1 then 5 mg/kg days 2–5) may hasten node resolution; most cases are self-limited.

5. Suspected TB/NTM lymphadenitis: do NOT start empiric antibiotics; obtain AFB smear/culture ± PCR; refer to ID/public health.

6. Toxoplasmosis with significant symptoms: consider pyrimethamine-sulfadiazine-leucovorin (specialist).

7. If abscess on US or fluctuance → incision & drainage ± culture; tailor antibiotics accordingly.

C. PROCEDURES

1. Needle aspiration for diagnostic culture in suppurative nodes (esp. children) if trained; otherwise refer for I&D.
2. Arrange excisional biopsy for persistent (>4–6 wks), enlarging, or high-risk nodes; coordinate with ENT/ general surgery; send for histology, flow cytometry, and cultures (including AFB).

DISPOSITION (DISCHARGE/OBSERVE/ TRANSFER) & RETURN PRECAUTIONS

1. Discharge with plan when stable: observation vs targeted antibiotics; schedule re-exam in 2–4 wks (earlier if antibiotics started).
2. Urgent referral: supraclavicular nodes; hard/fixed nodes; persistent >2 cm beyond 4–6 wks; generalized adenopathy; B-symptoms; abnormal CBC (cytopenias/ blasts) or CXR; airway symptoms; suspected TB/NTM.
3. ED/Immediate: airway compromise (stridor, drooling), rapidly enlarging tender mass with systemic toxicity (deep neck space infection), severe dehydration, sepsis.
4. Return immediately for: worsening swelling/pain, fever, dysphagia/voice change, breathing difficulty, new bruising/bleeding, weight loss/night sweats.

PEARLS & PITFALLS

1. Location matters: supraclavicular nodes are malignant until proven otherwise; epitrochlear/popliteal nodes are uncommon and warrant evaluation.

2. Do not over-treat post-viral nodes with antibiotics; most resolve. Re-examine instead.

3. Avoid corticosteroids before biopsy when lymphoma is on the table — can obscure diagnosis.

4. Ultrasound is first line for pediatric neck masses and to assess for abscess; CT/MRI reserved for complications or malignancy concern.

5. Think dental/skin sources; inspect scalp, oral cavity, and teeth for infections that drain to the involved basin.

REFERENCES

1. AAFP. Unexplained Lymphadenopathy: Evaluation and Differential Diagnosis (open). aafp.org

2. NICE CKS. Lymphadenopathy — assessment and management (public). cks.nice.org.uk

3. Royal Children's Hospital (Melbourne). Clinical Practice Guidelines: Cervical lymphadenopathy (open). rch.org.au

4. CDC. Bartonella (Cat Scratch Disease) — clinical overview; Epstein-Barr Virus; Tuberculosis resources (public). cdc.gov

5. Cancer Research UK / NICE NG12. Suspected cancer: recognition and referral (nodes and neck masses) (open). nice.org.uk; cancerresearchuk.org

6. IDSA/ATS public materials on TB diagnosis and management (open summaries). idsociety.org / thoracic.org

7. DermNet NZ. Lymphadenopathy overview and related infections (public). dermnetnz.org

LYMPHOMA VS LEUKEMIA, MULTIPLE MYELOMA, MGUS

OVERVIEW & "DON'T MISS"

1. Hematologic malignancies may present subtly in primary care. Think in 4 buckets: lymphoma (nodal/ extra-nodal masses), leukemia (circulating/ marrow disease), plasma-cell disorders (MM/MGUS), and reactive mimics.

2. Key clinical contrasts:

3. Lymphoma — painless, persistent lymphadenopathy ± 'B' symptoms (fever, drenching night sweats, weight loss), pruritus, mediastinal mass (HL).

4. Leukemia — fatigue/infections/bleeding due to cytopenias; splenomegaly; very high or very low WBC; blasts (acute) or mature lymphocytosis (CLL).

5. Multiple myeloma — 'CRAB' features: hyperCalcemia, Renal impairment, Anemia, Bone pain/lytic Bone lesions; recurrent infections, hyperviscosity, neuropathy/amyloidosis.

6. MGUS — asymptomatic monoclonal protein without CRAB/myeloma-defining events; requires risk-based

monitoring.

7. DON'T MISS: spinal cord compression/plasmacytoma (back pain + neuro deficits), hypercalcemic crisis, sepsis or neutropenic fever, tumor lysis (rare de novo), SVC syndrome, symptomatic hyperviscosity (headache/visual changes, epistaxis).

HISTORY & EXAM

1. Timeline: persistent nodes (>4–6 wks), constitutional symptoms; bone/back/rib pain; bruising/bleeding; infections; pruritus; abdominal fullness (splenomegaly); neuropathy; urinary symptoms (renal impairment).

2. Risk factors: age >50 (MM/CLL), family history, autoimmune disease/immune suppression (post-transplant), chronic infections (H. pylori, HBV/HCV, HIV), prior chemo/radiation, occupational exposures.

3. Examination: node survey (size/site/consistency; supraclavicular high-risk), spleen/liver size, skin (bruises/petechiae, rashes), oropharynx (tonsillar asymmetry), chest (mediastinal signs), spine tenderness, neuro exam (cord compression), performance status.

DIFFERENTIAL DIAGNOSIS (TOP 5)

1. Reactive lymphadenopathy (viral, bacterial incl. dental/skin, TB/NTM).

2. Autoimmune/inflammatory (sarcoidosis, SLE).

3. Solid-organ malignancy with nodal metastasis (H&N, lung, GI, GU, melanoma).

4. Hematologic malignancies: HL/NHL, CLL/CML/ALL/ AML.

5. Plasma-cell dyscrasias: MGUS, smoldering MM, overt multiple myeloma, AL amyloidosis.

INVESTIGATIONS (POC/LABS/IMAGING)

1. Initial labs (office/urgent): CBC with differential & smear (blasts, smudge cells), CMP (Ca/Cr/LFTs), LDH, uric acid, CRP/ESR. Consider beta-2 microglobulin (if accessible).

2. Myeloma pathway: SPEP with immunofixation, serum free light chains (κ/λ and ratio), ± UPEP/24-h urine protein with immunofixation if monoclonal band; quantify total protein/albumin gap. If screen positive or high suspicion → urgent hematology; imaging for bone disease (low-dose whole-body CT preferred; if unavailable, skeletal survey; MRI for focal symptoms).

3. Lymphoma pathway: ultrasound of accessible nodes; avoid steroids before biopsy. Excisional node biopsy is preferred for suspected lymphoma; core/FNA less sensitive for lymphoma typing.

4. Leukemia pathway: if blasts or cytopenias with systemic symptoms — SAME-DAY hematology/ED. Peripheral blood flow cytometry can diagnose CLL in persistent lymphocytosis (ALC $\geq 5 \times 10^9$/L for ≥ 3 months).

5. Infectious/secondary causes as indicated: HIV, HBV/HCV, TB testing, H. pylori (MALT features), autoimmune screen if suggestive.

6. Imaging for red flags: CXR if mediastinal mass/resp symptoms; urgent MRI spine if back pain + neuro deficits/sphincter symptoms.

MANAGEMENT (NON-PHARM → MEDS → PROCEDURES)

A. NON-PHARMACOLOGIC

1. Immediate safety-netting: written red-flag list (fever ≥38.0°C, rigors, bleeding, rapidly enlarging node/ mass, new neuro deficits, severe bone pain, confusion, anuria/oliguria).

2. Vaccinations: influenza, COVID-19, pneumococcal, and shingles (RZV) as appropriate prior to immunosuppressive therapy; avoid live vaccines once on significant immunosuppression.

3. Analgesia and fall-risk measures for bone pain; avoid high-impact activity if lytic lesions suspected until imaging completed.

B. MEDICATIONS (EXAMPLES; PRIMARY-CARE SCOPE — INDIVIDUALIZE)

1. Do NOT start corticosteroids if lymphoma/leukemia suspected without specialist input — can obscure diagnosis.

2. Hypercalcemia (suspected myeloma): hydrate with

oral/IV fluids; stop thiazides/lithium; avoid NSAIDs in CKD; urgent hematology/ED if Ca markedly elevated or symptomatic; bisphosphonates are specialist-initiated.

3. Infection prophylaxis is specialist-directed; however, counsel early care-seeking for fever and consider same-day evaluation if neutropenia suspected.

4. Anemia symptomatic: evaluate and correct reversible causes (iron/B12/folate, CKD). Transfusion decisions and disease-directed therapy are specialist-led.

C. PROCEDURES

1. Arrange urgent excisional node biopsy via surgery/ ENT for suspected lymphoma; ensure pathology requests include flow cytometry and microbiology (AFB) if indicated.

2. Order/coordinate SPEP/UPEP and serum free light chains when myeloma suspected; discuss imaging modality availability (low-dose WB-CT vs skeletal survey) with hematology.

3. For persistent lymphocytosis suggestive of CLL, request peripheral blood flow cytometry and LDH; arrange hematology referral.

DISPOSITION (DISCHARGE/OBSERVE/ TRANSFER) & RETURN PRECAUTIONS

1. Immediate ED/transfer: suspected acute leukemia (blasts with cytopenias or symptomatic

hyperleukocytosis), cord compression, SVC syndrome, hypercalcemic crisis, severe anemia with instability, tumor lysis signs (AKI, K$^+\uparrow$, phosphate$\uparrow$), neutropenic fever, symptomatic hyperviscosity (vision change, headache, mucosal bleeding).

2. Urgent (days) hematology: persistent unexplained lymphadenopathy (>2 cm, >4–6 wks), B-symptoms, unexplained cytopenias, ALC ≥5×10^9/L for ≥3 months, positive monoclonal protein with symptoms or abnormal FLC ratio, elevated Ca/Cr/anemia with bone pain.

3. Follow-up (weeks): low-risk MGUS without red flags after baseline risk stratification and education (see below).

PEARLS & PITFALLS

1. Unexplained back/rib pain + anemia + elevated total protein/'protein gap' → think myeloma; order SPEP and FLC early.

2. Avoid attributing persistent lymphadenopathy to 'reactive' without re-exam; supraclavicular nodes are malignant until proven otherwise.

3. MGUS criteria (common): M-protein <3 g/dL (30 g/L), marrow clonal plasma cells <10%, and no CRAB/ myeloma-defining events. Risk of progression ≈1%/ yr; stratify by Mayo 3-factor model (non-IgG type, M-protein ≥1.5 g/dL, abnormal FLC ratio) to plan follow-up (e.g., 6 mo then yearly if low-risk).

4. CLL often presents with sustained lymphocytosis;

many are observed ('watch & wait') until symptomatic cytopenias, bulky nodes, or infections — management is hematology-led.

5. Do not delay referral waiting for every test — early specialist involvement improves time to diagnosis and therapy.

REFERENCES

1. NICE Guideline NG12. Suspected cancer: recognition and referral (hematologic sections; open). nice.org.uk

2. NCI (National Cancer Institute) PDQ® (open). Adult Non-Hodgkin Lymphoma; Hodgkin Lymphoma; CLL; Acute Leukemias; and Plasma Cell Neoplasms (Multiple Myeloma). cancer.gov

3. International Myeloma Foundation — Diagnostic criteria and patient/clinician resources (open). myeloma.org

4. American Cancer Society — Lymphoma, Leukemia, Multiple Myeloma overviews (open). cancer.org

5. AAFP. Multiple Myeloma: Recognition and Management; Unexplained Lymphadenopathy; Evaluation of Abnormal Lymphocytosis (open articles). aafp.org

6. NCCN Guidelines for Patients® (open access): CLL/ SLL, Multiple Myeloma, Lymphomas. nccn.org/patients

7. Cancer Research UK — Tests for myeloma and lymphoma; MGUS information (open). cancerresearchuk.org

DO NOT MISS CANCER — RED FLAGS IN FAMILY PRACTICE

OVERVIEW & "DON'T MISS"

1. Aim: recognize 'alarm' features early, investigate appropriately without delay, and refer via urgent cancer pathways.

2. General red flags: unexplained weight loss, persistent fatigue, new persistent pain, fevers/night sweats, anorexia, new/worsening lumps, persistent or unexplained bleeding, and unexplained iron-deficiency anemia.

3. DON'T MISS emergencies: spinal cord compression (back pain + neuro deficits), superior vena cava (SVC) syndrome, massive hemoptysis, hypercalcemic crisis, bowel obstruction, acute liver failure, neutropenic sepsis (post-chemo).

HISTORY & EXAM

1. Timeline & persistence (>3–6 weeks), progression, systemic symptoms (B-symptoms), exposures (smoking, alcohol, asbestos), family history (early or

multiple cancers), and prior abnormal screens.

2. Bleeding: postmenopausal bleeding; rectal bleeding with change in bowel habit; hemoptysis; hematuria (visible or non-visible).

3. GI: dysphagia/odynophagia; new dyspepsia >55 with weight loss; persistent change in bowel habit; jaundice (painless); abdominal mass.

4. Respiratory: cough >3 weeks (esp. >40 with smoking/occupational risks), chest pain, dyspnea, hoarseness >3 weeks.

5. Breast: new lump, skin dimpling, nipple inversion/discharge (bloody), eczematous nipple change; axillary nodes.

6. GU: visible hematuria; recurrent non-visible hematuria; persistent LUTS with abnormal DRE; testicular mass, heaviness, or pain.

7. Gyn: postmenopausal bleeding; intermenstrual/post-coital bleeding; persistent abdominal bloating/early satiety (ovarian).

8. Skin: evolving lesion (ABCDE for pigmented lesions), non-healing ulcer, pearly bleed-prone papule, rapidly growing nodules.

9. Neuro: new seizures, focal deficits, headaches worse on waking/with Valsalva; personality/cognitive change with subacute course.

10. Nodes: unexplained lymphadenopathy >6 weeks, hard/fixed/supraclavicular; generalized pruritus/night sweats.

DIFFERENTIAL DIAGNOSIS (TOP 5)

1. Infections (TB, endocarditis, chronic viral hepatitis, H. pylori) mimicking weight loss/fevers/anemia.

2. Benign GI/GU causes of bleeding (hemorrhoids, BPH) — still investigate age-appropriately.

3. Benign breast disease (cysts/fibroadenoma) — image per age/risk.

4. Autoimmune/inflammatory disease (IBD, vasculitis) and endocrine (thyroid) causing systemic symptoms.

5. Medication effects (anticoagulants causing bleeding, PPIs/NSAIDs causing dyspepsia) — do not attribute without evaluation.

INVESTIGATIONS (POC/LABS/IMAGING)

1. Do not delay urgent referral for tests that won't change triage; follow local 'suspected cancer' pathways (e.g., 2-week wait).

2. Basic labs: CBC (look for IDA, leukocytosis, thrombocytosis), ferritin/iron studies, CMP (LFTs incl. cholestatic vs hepatocellular pattern, calcium), CRP/ESR, urinalysis.

3. CXR for persistent cough/hemoptysis/unexplained weight loss (>40); ultrasound for persistent abdominal mass; pelvic US for postmenopausal bleeding (endometrial thickness).

4. FIT vs symptomatic: symptomatic rectal bleeding/change in habit generally warrant urgent colorectal assessment regardless of FIT; check local pathway.

5. Visible hematuria → urgent urology (cystoscopy + imaging). Non-visible hematuria persistent → urology, esp. age >60 or risk factors.

6. Breast: age-appropriate imaging (US ± diagnostic mammography).

7. Head & neck: urgent ENT for persistent hoarseness >3 weeks, oral ulcer >3 weeks, unilateral sore throat/ otalgia with normal ear exam, dysphagia, neck mass.

MANAGEMENT (NON-PHARM → MEDS → PROCEDURES)

A. NON-PHARMACOLOGIC

1. Immediate safety-netting: provide clear written return precautions (worsening bleeding, pain, neurologic symptoms, fever/rigors, inability to eat/drink).

2. Stop/avoid potential confounders: e.g., do not start steroids when lymphoma suspected (may obscure diagnosis); hold unnecessary iron before ferritin if feasible (do not delay care).

3. Risk factor modification: smoking cessation, alcohol reduction, weight management; update vaccinations (HPV, hep B).

B. MEDICATIONS (EXAMPLES; INDIVIDUALIZE)

1. Symptom relief while awaiting work-up: analgesia (acetaminophen ± short NSAID course if renal/GI safe), antiemetics, laxatives for obstructive symptoms (avoid if peritonitis/obstruction suspected).

2. Do not empirically treat with antibiotics or PPIs repeatedly for persistent red-flag symptoms without arranging definitive evaluation.

3. Iron deficiency anemia: start oral iron (alternate-day dosing) if symptomatic, but concurrently arrange source evaluation (men/postmenopausal women → GI until proven otherwise).

4. Anticoagulation: in unprovoked VTE, do standard treatment; extensive occult cancer CT screening generally not recommended beyond age-appropriate screening and targeted evaluation of symptoms/signs.

C. PROCEDURES

1. Urgent referrals: follow suspected cancer criteria by site (breast, colorectal, lung, urology, gyn, head & neck, hematology, derm).

2. Point-of-care: fecal occult blood/FIT (as per pathway), skin dermoscopy if trained, pelvic exam/speculum for bleeding, DRE for rectal/occult mass, lymph node exam with documentation and recheck in 2–6 weeks if low suspicion.

DISPOSITION (DISCHARGE/OBSERVE/ TRANSFER) & RETURN PRECAUTIONS

1. ED/Immediate transfer: suspected cord compression (new back pain with leg weakness/saddle anesthesia/ urinary retention), SVC syndrome (facial/arm swelling, dyspnea), massive hemoptysis, hypercalcemic crisis (confusion, dehydration, arrhythmia), bowel obstruction

(vomiting, obstipation, peritonitis), acute liver failure (jaundice + coagulopathy/encephalopathy).

2. Urgent referral (days): postmenopausal bleeding; visible hematuria; persistent hoarseness/dysphagia; oral ulcer/neck mass >3 weeks; breast lump or suspicious skin lesion; unexplained weight loss + GI symptoms; unexplained IDA; chronic cough/ hemoptysis; painless jaundice.

3. Safety-net: specific timeframe to re-review (usually 2–6 weeks). If symptoms persist/progress despite initial negative tests, escalate or seek second opinion.

PEARLS & PITFALLS

1. Three-visit rule: if the patient returns twice with persistent symptoms, escalate work-up/referral on the third visit.

2. Men or post-menopausal women with iron-deficiency anemia have GI cancer until proven otherwise — arrange bidirectional endoscopy unless another clear source exists.

3. Do not attribute rectal bleeding to hemorrhoids without appropriate evaluation in older adults.

4. Smokers >40 with persistent cough or weight loss → get a CXR and consider urgent assessment for lung cancer.

5. Postmenopausal bleeding is endometrial cancer until proven otherwise — urgent pelvic ultrasound/ endometrial assessment.

6. Avoid corticosteroids before tissue diagnosis when lymphoma or brain tumor is suspected (can obscure pathology).

7. Document safety-netting and give clear written return precautions.

REFERENCES

1. NICE Guideline NG12. Suspected cancer: recognition and referral (open). nice.org.uk

2. NICE Quality Standard QS124. Suspected cancer — urgent referral pathways (open). nice.org.uk

3. Cancer Research UK. Suspected cancer referral guidelines for GPs (open). cancerresearchuk.org

4. AAFP. Recognizing and Managing Red Flags for Cancer in Primary Care; Evaluating Unintentional Weight Loss (open articles). aafp.org

5. Canadian Task Force on Preventive Health Care & provincial 'Rapid Access Clinics' pages (open) — symptomatic pathways (varies by province).

6. American Cancer Society. Signs and Symptoms of Cancer — patient-facing, useful for safety-netting (open). cancer.org

7. Choosing Wisely Canada. Avoid repeated empirical treatment without evaluation of alarm symptoms (public). choosingwiselycanada.org

INFECTIOUS DISEASE / ENVIRONMENTAL

PID/TOA, STI SCREENING & TREATMENT, SEXUAL ASSAULT CARE

OVERVIEW & "DON'T MISS"

1. PID = ascending infection of upper genital tract; can lead to infertility, ectopic pregnancy, chronic pelvic pain.
2. TOA = PID complication with walled-off abscess; risk of rupture and sepsis.
3. DON'T MISS: ectopic pregnancy, appendicitis, ovarian torsion, ruptured TOA, septic shock; in sexual assault, immediate safety and consent-based care.

HISTORY & EXAM

1. Sexual history (5 Ps), recent partners, contraception, last intercourse, STI history, douching; assault: time since event, injuries, strangulation, weapon use, consent for exam/evidence.
2. Symptoms: pelvic/abdominal pain, fever, abnormal bleeding/discharge, dyspareunia, dysuria, N/V.
3. Exam: vitals; abdominal exam; pelvic exam (speculum + bimanual) if tolerated—look for cervical motion,

uterine/adnexal tenderness, masses; document injuries; trauma-informed approach.

DIFFERENTIAL DIAGNOSIS (TOP 5)

1. Ectopic pregnancy; ovarian torsion; appendicitis; UTI/ pyelonephritis; endometriosis/ruptured cyst.

INVESTIGATIONS (POC/LABS/IMAGING)

1. Pregnancy test (urine/serum) for all of reproductive potential.
2. NAAT for chlamydia/gonorrhea (cervical/vaginal or urine), and consider extragenital NAATs based on exposure; wet mount/POC for trichomonas if available.
3. HIV Ag/Ab, syphilis serology, HBsAg; consider HCV based on risk; urine dip/culture if urinary symptoms.
4. CBC, CRP if systemic illness; pelvic ultrasound when TOA, torsion, or ectopic suspected.
5. Sexual assault: offer forensic evidence collection where available (with consent); document carefully; follow local chain-of-custody protocols.

MANAGEMENT (NON-PHARM → MEDS → PROCEDURES)

A. NON-PHARMACOLOGIC

1. Trauma-informed care; obtain informed consent for each step; offer chaperone; manage pain promptly.
2. Abstain from sex until therapy complete and symptoms

resolved; counsel on partner notification and treatment; provide written instructions.

3. Link to community supports: sexual assault services, crisis lines, social work; safety planning as needed.

B. MEDICATIONS (EXAMPLES; CONFIRM LOCAL GUIDANCE)

1. Outpatient PID: ceftriaxone 500 mg IM once (1 g if ≥150 kg) + doxycycline 100 mg PO BID × 14 days + metronidazole 500 mg PO BID × 14 days.

2. Inpatient PID/TOA or severe disease: start IV broad-spectrum (e.g., ceftriaxone 1 g IV q24h + doxycycline 100 mg IV/PO BID + metronidazole 500 mg IV/PO BID; OR cefoxitin 2 g IV q6h + doxycycline; OR clindamycin + gentamicin). Step down to complete 14 days total once improved.

3. TOA: urgent gynecology consult; consider IR/surgical drainage if large (≈ ≥7–8 cm) or not improving within 48–72 h.

4. STI treatment highlights (adults, uncomplicated): chlamydia — doxycycline 100 mg PO BID × 7 days; gonorrhea — ceftriaxone 500 mg IM once (1 g if ≥150 kg) + doxycycline if chlamydia not excluded; trichomoniasis — metronidazole 2 g PO once or 500 mg PO BID × 7 days; syphilis — benzathine penicillin G dosing per stage; treat partners per guidelines.

5. Sexual assault prophylaxis bundle (offer, with consent): empiric STI prophylaxis (ceftriaxone + doxycycline + metronidazole), emergency

contraception (copper IUD up to 5 days or ulipristal 30 mg up to 5 days), hepatitis B vaccine ± HBIG if non-immune, HPV vaccine if eligible, HIV PEP if risk within 72 h; tetanus update if indicated.

C. PROCEDURES

1. IUD for emergency contraception (copper) if desired and no contraindication; ultrasound-guided aspiration/ drainage for TOA when indicated; follow local forensic protocols for evidence collection.

DISPOSITION (DISCHARGE/OBSERVE/ TRANSFER) & RETURN PRECAUTIONS

1. Discharge (most mild–moderate PID): start therapy, provide partner management and safety-netting; re-evaluate in 48–72 h; retest for STIs in ~3 months.

2. Observe/urgent same-day: intolerance of PO meds, high fever, diagnostic uncertainty, early pregnancy, or inadequate home support.

3. Admit/Transfer: suspected TOA/rupture, severe illness/ sepsis, pregnancy, surgical emergencies (torsion/ appendicitis), failure to improve in 48–72 h, or inability to ensure follow-up.

4. Return immediately for: worsening pain/fever, syncope, persistent vomiting, new focal peritonitis, pregnancy symptoms after assault, chest pain/SOB, severe headache/neurologic deficits.

PEARLS & PITFALLS

1. Low threshold to treat PID when pelvic tenderness + STI risk — early treatment reduces sequelae.

2. Consider extragenital testing (pharyngeal/rectal) based on exposures; treat partners promptly.

3. Avoid digital vaginal exam before speculum when concern for bleeding/trauma; in assault cases, prioritize consent and documentation quality.

4. Re-dose ceftriaxone for weight ≥150 kg; review medication allergies and pregnancy status before therapy.

5. Schedule follow-up testing and offer vaccinations (HBV/HPV); ensure access to HIV PEP where indicated.

REFERENCES

1. Public Health Agency of Canada (PHAC). Canadian Guidelines on Sexually Transmitted Infections — PID, chlamydia, gonorrhea, syphilis, trichomoniasis. Public: canada.ca

2. BC Centre for Disease Control (BCCDC). STI Treatment Guidelines (public). Public: bccdc.ca

3. U.S. CDC. 2021 STI Treatment Guidelines — PID, chlamydia, gonorrhea, sexual assault clinical considerations (online, public). Public: cdc.gov/std/treatment

4. BASHH (UK). PID Guideline (public). Public: bashh.org

5. NICE. Pelvic inflammatory disease: diagnosis and management (public). Public: nice.org.uk

6. WHO. Clinical management of rape and intimate partner violence survivors (public). Public: who.int

7. SAFEta / U.S. DOJ. National Protocol for Sexual Assault Medical Forensic Examinations (public). Public: safeta.org

ANIMAL BITES — FAMILY MEDICINE OFFICE (DOG/CAT/HUMAN/WILDLIFE)

OVERVIEW & "DON'T MISS"

1. High infection risk wounds: cat bites (deep punctures, Pasteurella), hand bites, crush injuries, delayed presentation (>12 h extremity/>24 h face), immunocompromised/asplenic, penetrating joints/ tendons.

2. DON'T MISS: test/repair neurovascular/tendon injury, open joint/tenosynovitis, compartment syndrome, retained foreign body/teeth, osteomyelitis, septic arthritis, Capnocytophaga sepsis (asplenic, liver disease), rabies exposure, tetanus-prone wounds.

HISTORY & EXAM

1. Animal (species/breed), provoked vs unprovoked, domesticated/vaccinated vs stray/wild, availability for 10-day observation (dogs/cats/ferrets), geographic location/travel, indoor bat exposure.

2. Time since bite, first aid done, pain/swelling/fever, functional deficit; dominant hand; occupation;

immunization history (tetanus, rabies pre-exposure).

3. Risk conditions: asplenia, cirrhosis, diabetes, immunosuppression, prosthetic joints/valves, lymphedema.

4. Exam: size/depth, devitalized tissue, crush, puncture vs laceration, involvement of face/hand/genitals, proximity to joint/tendon sheath, neurovascular status; look for retained tooth fragments; regional nodes.

DIFFERENTIAL DIAGNOSIS (TOP 5)

1. Uncomplicated soft-tissue bite wound.

2. Cellulitis/abscess (Pasteurella multocida in cats; Staph/Strep; Capnocytophaga canimorsus in dogs).

3. Flexor tenosynovitis/septic arthritis/osteomyelitis after penetrating bite (hand highest risk).

4. Human bite ('fight bite') with Eikenella corrodens and mixed anaerobes.

5. Rabies exposure (dogs/cats/wild carnivores/bats) or tetanus-prone wound.

INVESTIGATIONS (POC/LABS/IMAGING)

1. Usually clinical. Consider X-ray for suspected foreign body (tooth), fracture, or periosteal involvement; hand bites near MCP ('fight bite') need careful imaging and exploration.

2. Baseline labs if systemic signs or high-risk (CBC, CRP). Blood cultures if septic. Joint aspiration if suspected septic arthritis.

3. Swab cultures are low yield; culture pus/tissue if draining or after debridement; obtain cultures before antibiotics for established infection.

MANAGEMENT (NON-PHARM → MEDS → PROCEDURES)

A. WOUND CARE (CORNERSTONE)

1. Immediate irrigation: copious high-pressure saline (≥500–1000 mL for moderate wounds); remove foreign material; conservative debridement of devitalized tissue.
2. Leave most puncture wounds (esp. cats) and hand/ foot bites open; primary closure acceptable for low-risk facial/scalp wounds after meticulous irrigation + prophylactic antibiotics.
3. Immobilize and elevate involved limb; ensure tetanus and rabies risk assessment before discharge.

B. ANTIBIOTICS (PROPHYLAXIS VS TREATMENT)

1. Prophylaxis (3–5 days) for: cat bites, hand bites, deep puncture/crush, through-and-through oral lacerations, delayed presentation, immunocompromised/asplenia, wounds near joint/tendon sheath.
2. First-line (adults): amoxicillin-clavulanate 875/125 mg PO BID (or 500/125 mg TID).
3. Penicillin allergy (non-anaphylactic): doxycycline 100 mg PO BID ± metronidazole 500 mg PO TID (adds anaerobic coverage).

4. Penicillin anaphylaxis or need single agent: moxifloxacin 400 mg PO daily (adults, non-pregnant).

5. Alternatives: TMP-SMX DS BID + metronidazole 500 mg TID; or clindamycin 300 mg QID + ciprofloxacin 500 mg BID (note: Eikenella is resistant to clindamycin/macrolides/1st-gen cephs).

6. Established infection: 5–7 days (cellulitis) or longer for tenosynovitis/septic arthritis/osteomyelitis (consult surgery/ID). IV options: ampicillin-sulbactam 3 g IV q6h; or ceftriaxone + metronidazole; piperacillin-tazobactam if severe.

7. Human bites ('fight bite'): ALWAYS prophylax/ treat; cover Eikenella and anaerobes (amox-clav or ampicillin-sulbactam).

C. RABIES POST-EXPOSURE PROPHYLAXIS (PEP)

1. Wound cleansing with soap and water + povidone-iodine as available reduces risk.

2. Assess exposure: dogs/cats/ferrets that remain healthy for 10 days after the bite were not infectious at the time; wild carnivores/bats generally indicate PEP unless animal tests negative; consider public health guidance.

3. PEP (not previously vaccinated): human rabies immune globulin (HRIG) 20 IU/kg — infiltrate as much as anatomically possible in/around wounds; remainder IM at site distant from vaccine. PLUS vaccine (1 mL IM in deltoid; anterolateral thigh for small children) on

days 0, 3, 7, 14 (add day 28 if immunocompromised).

4. Previously vaccinated: NO HRIG; give vaccine days 0 and 3 only.

5. Avoid gluteal injection for vaccine; do not mix HRIG and vaccine in same syringe/site.

D. TETANUS PROPHYLAXIS

1. Give Tdap/Td if ≥10 years since last dose (clean minor wounds) or ≥5 years for dirty/major wounds.

2. TIG (tetanus immune globulin) for dirty wounds if uncertain/incomplete primary series or severe immunodeficiency.

E. PROCEDURES/REFERRAL

1. Hand bites, suspected joint penetration, tendon sheath involvement (Kanavel signs), face wounds needing layered repair, large tissue loss, or delayed/infected wounds → surgical/hand/plastic consult.

2. Explore clenched-fist injuries over MCP with finger in flexion; copious irrigation; often require OR washout.

3. Imaging for foreign body/tooth; remove under adequate anesthesia; consider dental consult for tooth injury.

DISPOSITION (DISCHARGE/OBSERVE/ TRANSFER) & RETURN PRECAUTIONS

1. Immediate ED/transfer: systemic toxicity/sepsis, rapidly progressive cellulitis, severe hand infections/

tenosynovitis, suspected septic arthritis/osteomyelitis, compartment syndrome, uncontrolled bleeding.

2. Outpatient with close follow-up (24–48 h) for high-risk locations (hand/face/genitals) or immunocompromised.

3. Return immediately for: increasing pain/swelling/ erythema, fever, purulent drainage, red streaking, decreased ROM/sensation, new numbness/tingling, or inability to tolerate PO/medication.

PEARLS & PITFALLS

1. Amoxicillin alone, clindamycin alone, and 1st-gen cephalosporins are inadequate for cat/human bites.

2. Do not primarily close cat puncture or hand bites unless exceptional circumstances with prophylaxis.

3. Asplenic/cirrhotic patients are at risk for fulminant Capnocytophaga sepsis after dog bites — treat promptly and monitor closely.

4. Bat exposures can be subtle; if a bat is found in a room with a sleeping/unattended person, consult public health regarding PEP.

5. Document animal details and report to public health/ animal control per local law; consider rabies testing of the animal when feasible.

REFERENCES

1. CDC. Rabies: Post-exposure prophylaxis & animal management; Tetanus: wound management (public). cdc.gov

2. WHO. Rabies post-exposure prophylaxis guidance (open). who.int

3. NICE CKS. Bites — human and animal; Tetanus (public). cks.nice.org.uk

4. AAFP. Dog and Cat Bites: Evaluation and Management; Prevention and Treatment of Animal Bites (open articles). aafp.org

5. IDSA. 2014 Skin and Soft Tissue Infections Guideline — animal/human bite sections (open summary). idsociety.org

6. Public Health Agency resources (country/province/state) on rabies risk assessment and PEP algorithms (public).

TRAVEL MEDICINE

OVERVIEW & "DON'T MISS"

1. Pre-travel consult: risk assessment (destination, itinerary, timing/season, activities, accommodations), vaccines, malaria risk/chemoprophylaxis, traveler's diarrhea (TD) strategy, injury prevention, insurance, documentation.

2. Post-travel: any fever in the first year after travel to malaria-endemic areas is malaria until ruled out.

3. DON'T MISS: febrile illness after malaria-risk travel; severe dehydration from TD; hemorrhagic symptoms; respiratory distress; animal bites (rabies exposure); VTE after long flights; high-altitude illness; yellow fever vaccine contraindications.

HISTORY & EXAM

1. Itinerary (countries/regions, urban vs rural), dates/season, duration, layovers; purpose (tourism, VFR, humanitarian, business), accommodations (hostel, friends/family).

2. Activities/exposures: freshwater (schistosomiasis), animals (rabies), insects (malaria, dengue, Zika),

food/water hygiene, sexual exposures; altitude plans; diving; adventure/road travel.

3. Medical: pregnancy/intent, immunosuppression, chronic disease, allergies, prior vaccine reactions; meds (anticoagulants), G6PD status if considering primaquine/tafenoquine.

4. Exam: vitals, general exam; focused exam if post-travel ill (rash, eschar, jaundice, dehydration, lungs, neuro).

DIFFERENTIAL DIAGNOSIS (TOP 5)

1. Malaria (any fever within 1 year after risk exposure).

2. Dengue/chikungunya/Zika (Aedes areas).

3. Traveler's diarrhea (ETEC/EAEC/Campylobacter, etc.).

4. Typhoid/paratyphoid fever (enteric fever).

5. Acute mountain sickness vs. viral URI (if altitude exposure).

INVESTIGATIONS (POC/LABS/IMAGING)

1. Pre-travel: generally none; review immunization records. Consider pregnancy test if giving live vaccines; G6PD for primaquine/tafenoquine when indicated.

2. Post-travel fever: malaria smears/rapid test URGENT (repeat x3 if negative and suspicion persists); CBC (leukopenia/thrombocytopenia), LFTs, blood cultures, urinalysis; stool studies for persistent diarrhea (ova/parasites, Giardia/Crypto antigen).

3. Altitude illness: pulse oximetry if available; otherwise clinical diagnosis.

MANAGEMENT (NON-PHARM → MEDS → PROCEDURES)

A. NON-PHARMACOLOGIC

1. Food/water safety: 'boil it, cook it, peel it, or forget it'; safe beverages (sealed, treated); hand hygiene.

2. Insect bite prevention: 20–30% DEET or 20% icaridin/ picaridin; permethrin-treated clothing/bed nets; dawn/ dusk precautions; Aedes are day-biters.

3. Altitude: gradual ascent; sleep low; rest day every 600–900 m above 3000 m; avoid alcohol/sedatives; recognize AMS/HACE/HAPE signs.

4. Flights/DVT: move q1–2 h, calf exercises, aisle seat, hydration; compression stockings if high-risk.

5. Insurance & documents: travel medical/evac insurance; carry vaccine proofs (e.g., yellow fever ICVP where required).

B. MEDICATIONS (EXAMPLES; INDIVIDUALIZE TO DESTINATION/RESISTANCE/PATIENT FACTORS)

1. Malaria chemoprophylaxis (choose ONE based on destination/resistance, renal/hepatic function, pregnancy, price):

2. Atovaquone-proguanil 250/100 mg PO daily — start 1–2 days before, during travel, continue 7 days after;

avoid in severe renal impairment.

3. Doxycycline 100 mg PO daily — start 1–2 days before, during, continue 4 weeks after; photosensitivity/ esophagitis; avoid in pregnancy/young children.

4. Mefloquine 250 mg PO weekly — start ≥2 weeks before, during, continue 4 weeks after; contraindications include certain neuropsychiatric/ cardiac disorders; may be preferred in pregnancy if effective region.

5. Chloroquine 300 mg base weekly where sensitive (limited regions).

6. Traveler's diarrhea self-care: oral rehydration; loperamide for non-bloody diarrhea; consider bismuth subsalicylate. Antibiotics for severe/moderate dysentery or disabling illness:

7. Azithromycin 1 g PO once or 500 mg PO daily × 1–3 days (preferred in South/Southeast Asia).

8. Ciprofloxacin 750 mg once or 500 mg BID × 3 days (avoid where resistance high; avoid in pregnancy/ children).

9. Rifaximin 200 mg TID × 3 days for non-invasive disease (not for dysentery/fever).

10. Altitude: acetazolamide 125 mg PO BID (prophylaxis) starting 24h before ascent, continue 48h at altitude or until descent; treatment 250 mg PO BID. Dexamethasone 4 mg PO/IM/IV q6h as rescue for severe AMS/HACE (does not aid acclimatization).

11. Jet lag: short-course melatonin 0.5–3 mg at

destination bedtime; timed light exposure; sleep schedule adjustments.

12. Rabies: prompt wound irrigation; consider pre-exposure vaccine (2-dose day 0 and 7 schedule per ACIP) for high-risk itineraries; ensure PEP access planning in remote areas.

C. PROCEDURES

1. Administer indicated vaccines: routine updates (Tdap, MMR, varicella), Hep A, Hep B, Typhoid (Vi IM single dose or Ty21a oral days 0,2,4,6), Yellow fever (ICVP documentation; live vaccine contraindications: severe immunosuppression, age <6 months; caution in >60 yrs), Japanese encephalitis (0, 28 days), cholera (per indication), meningococcal (e.g., Hajj/Umrah requirement).

2. Provide written plan: malaria regimen, TD antibiotics, altitude strategy, emergency contacts; assemble travel kit (ORS, antipyretics, loperamide, insect repellent, condoms, basic wound care).

DISPOSITION (DISCHARGE/OBSERVE/ TRANSFER) & RETURN PRECAUTIONS

1. Pre-travel: discharge with vaccines given, prescriptions, and clear instructions; schedule follow-up if multi-dose series.

2. Post-travel illness: ED referral for fever in malaria-risk traveler, severe dehydration, respiratory distress, neuro symptoms, or bleeding.

3. Return urgently for: fever, bloody diarrhea, jaundice, severe headache, confusion, SOB, chest pain, oliguria; after animal bite/scratch, seek care immediately for PEP.

PEARLS & PITFALLS

1. 'Fever + travel' = malaria rule-out priority — don't delay testing for lack of classic periodic fevers.
2. VFR (visiting friends and relatives) travelers have higher risk and often present late — prioritize outreach and accelerated schedules.
3. Live vaccines: avoid in pregnancy and severe immunosuppression; separate live-live by ≥4 weeks if not same day.
4. Avoid co-administration of doxycycline with antacids/iron; photosensitivity counselling.
5. Document lot numbers and provide International Certificate of Vaccination when required.

REFERENCES

1. WHO. International Travel and Health (ITH) — country pages, vaccine recommendations, malaria, yellow fever certificates. Public: who.int
2. CDC. Yellow Book (online) — malaria prophylaxis, traveler's diarrhea, altitude illness, jet lag. Public: cdc.gov/yellowbook
3. CATMAT (PHAC). Canadian recommendations for the prevention and treatment of travel-related infections

(malaria, JE, rabies, cholera, travelers' diarrhea).
Public: canada.ca

4. Government of Canada — Travel health notices &
destination advice. Public: travel.gc.ca

5. NaTHNaC / TravelHealthPro (UK) — country
vaccine recommendations and disease risks. Public:
travelhealthpro.org.uk

6. NACI (PHAC) — Statements: Tdap in pregnancy,
COVID-19, influenza, hepatitis, zoster; Yellow fever &
JE guidance. Public: canada.ca

7. Fit for Travel (NHS Scotland) — public country
vaccination guidance. Public: fitfortravel.nhs.uk

VACCINES — ADULT & PEDIATRIC (TRAVEL WHEN APPLICABLE)

OVERVIEW & "DON'T MISS"

1. Routine immunization prevents severe morbidity/ mortality across the lifespan; use age-based schedules plus risk-based indications (chronic disease, pregnancy, immunocompromise, occupational/travel).

2. DON'T MISS: anaphylaxis (ABC, epinephrine IM 0.01 mg/kg up to 0.5 mg; observe all patients ≥15 minutes—30 minutes if prior reactions); syncope with injury risk; vaccine storage excursions; live-vaccine contraindications (pregnancy, severe immunodeficiency).

3. For travel: assess itinerary, timing (≥4–6 weeks ideally), vaccines (routine + destination-specific), malaria/other chemoprophylaxis, and documentation (e.g., yellow fever card).

HISTORY & EXAM

1. Immunization history (childhood/adult), previous reactions, allergy (esp. anaphylaxis), pregnancy

status/intent, immunocompromise (disease/meds), asplenia, chronic conditions (cardiac, pulmonary, renal, hepatic, diabetes), occupation (HCW), living situation (LTCH), indigenous status, and travel plans.

2. Vitals as indicated; defer vaccination if moderate–severe acute illness with fever (minor illness is not a contraindication). Check temperature monitors if cold-chain concerns.

DIFFERENTIAL DIAGNOSIS (TOP 5)

1. Immediate allergic reaction vs. vasovagal syncope vs. anxiety/panic.
2. Local cellulitis vs. expected local reactogenicity (pain/redness/swelling).
3. Viral exanthem vs. vaccine-related rash (e.g., mild post-MMR).
4. Fever from intercurrent infection vs. expected transient post-vaccine fever.
5. Brachial neuritis/shoulder injury related to vaccine administration (SIRVA) vs. routine soreness.

INVESTIGATIONS (POC/LABS/IMAGING)

1. Generally none required. Serology selectively for uncertain immunity (e.g., hep B, varicella) or occupational requirements.
2. Pregnancy test if uncertainty prior to live vaccines; TB testing timing with live vaccines (same day or ≥4 weeks apart).

3. Travel: check destination-specific requirements (e.g., yellow fever) and timing constraints.

MANAGEMENT (NON-PHARM → MEDS → PROCEDURES)

A. NON-PHARMACOLOGIC

1. Use provincial/NACI schedules; offer opportunistic catch-up at every visit; address vaccine hesitancy with empathic, evidence-based dialogue.
2. Education: common reactions, when to seek care; avoid routine prophylactic antipyretics (may blunt immune response) but treat fever/discomfort if needed.
3. Cold-chain: maintain 2–8 °C; document lot/expiry/site/ route; complete public registry entries; report AEFIs to public health.

B. MEDICATIONS / VACCINES (EXAMPLES; FOLLOW CURRENT NACI/ACIP)

1. Pediatric core: HepB; DTaP-IPV-Hib; pneumococcal (PCV); rotavirus (age limits apply); MMR; varicella; Men-C/C-ACYW per program; influenza annually; COVID-19 per NACI; HPV starting age 9–12 (2-dose).
2. Adult core: Td/Tdap (1x Tdap, then Td/Tdap q10y); influenza annually; COVID-19 per NACI; pneumococcal (PCV20 or PCV15→PPSV23 per guidance for ≥65 or risk); shingles (recombinant zoster, 2 doses ≥50 or immunocompromised ≥18); HPV catch-up through age 26 (consider to 45); hepatitis A/B

for risk groups; meningococcal for indications; MMR/varicella if non-immune.

3. Pregnancy: inactivated influenza any trimester; Tdap at 27–32 weeks each pregnancy; avoid live vaccines (MMR, varicella, live-attenuated influenza, yellow fever unless risk outweighs).

4. Immunocompromise/asplenia: ensure PCV/PPSV, Men-ACYW + MenB, Hib adult dose (asplenia), HepA/B as indicated; avoid live vaccines per degree of immunosuppression.

5. Travel (examples; verify CATMAT/CDC/WHO): hepatitis A; typhoid; yellow fever (where required/indicated); Japanese encephalitis (specific Asia/Pacific exposures); cholera (limited indications); rabies pre-exposure for high-risk. Documentations and intervals vary.

C. PROCEDURES

1. Administration: IM (deltoid ≥12 mo; anterolateral thigh in infants); SC for MMR/varicella (per product); anatomic landmarking to avoid SIRVA.

2. Spacing: inactivated vaccines can be co-administered; live-live same day or ≥4 weeks apart; post-IVIG timing for live vaccines per NACI tables.

3. Observation: ≥15 minutes; manage syncope safety; ensure epinephrine kit ready.

DISPOSITION (DISCHARGE/OBSERVE/ TRANSFER) & RETURN PRECAUTIONS

1. Discharge with after-care sheet and next-dose schedule; arrange recalls (EMR reminders/registries).

2. Observe/urgent review: worsening local reaction with fever after 24–48 h (cellulitis), persistent high fever, or concerning systemic symptoms.

3. Transfer/ED: suspected anaphylaxis, respiratory compromise, hypotension, neurologic deficits.

PEARLS & PITFALLS

1. Use single-visit co-administration to improve completion; don't delay for minor illness.

2. Check product-specific age limits (e.g., rotavirus maximum age), and dose volumes/routes.

3. Document lot/expiry/site/route and provide an updated record; enroll in provincial registries where available.

4. Live vaccines: avoid in pregnancy; counsel on contraception window after MMR/varicella (typically 1 month).

5. For yellow fever or other live travel vaccines in pregnancy or severe immunosuppression, seek specialist advice and consider waivers where appropriate.

REFERENCES

1. Public Health Agency of Canada (PHAC). Canadian Immunization Guide (CIG) — schedules,

contraindications, storage, and vaccine-specific chapters. Public: canada.ca

2. NACI (PHAC). Statements and updates for influenza, COVID-19, pneumococcal, zoster, HPV, Tdap in pregnancy, etc. Public: canada.ca

3. Government of Saskatchewan. Routine immunization schedules (infant/child/adult) and publicly funded programs. Public: saskatchewan.ca / saskhealthauthority.ca

4. CDC/ACIP. Child/Adolescent and Adult Immunization Schedules (with job aids). Public: cdc.gov

5. WHO. International travel and health; vaccine position papers; country vaccine requirements (e.g., yellow fever). Public: who.int

6. CATMAT (PHAC). Canadian recommendations for the prevention and treatment of travel-related infections (e.g., yellow fever, JE, rabies, cholera, typhoid). Public: canada.ca

7. BC Centre for Disease Control & BC Immunization Manual (public sections). Public: bccdc.ca

NEUROLOGY

POST-CONCUSSION (MILD TRAUMATIC BRAIN INJURY) — FAMILY MEDICINE OFFICE

OVERVIEW & "DON'T MISS"

1. Concussion (mTBI) = transient disturbance of brain function after head/neck/rotational force. Typical symptoms: headache, dizziness, nausea, fogginess, sensitivity to light/noise, sleep and mood changes.

2. Most recover within 2–4 weeks; a subset develop persistent post-concussive symptoms (PPCS).

3. DON'T MISS (RED FLAGS → ED/CT pathway): worsening severe headache, repeated vomiting, seizure, focal neuro deficits, unequal pupils, confusion/agitation, GCS <15 two hours post-injury, anticoagulant/antiplatelet use with head trauma, skull fracture signs, neck pain with neuro deficits, intoxication masking exam.

HISTORY & EXAM

1. Mechanism and immediate symptoms (LOC, amnesia, confusion, ataxia); red flags; anticoagulants; prior

concussions; migraine/anxiety/ADHD/sleep disorders (risk for prolonged recovery).

2. Symptom inventory at baseline and follow-ups (e.g., SCAT6/Child SCAT6 checklists).

3. Focused neuro exam: mental status, cranial nerves (smooth pursuit/saccades), vestibular-ocular (VOMS), gait/balance (tandem, single-leg), cervical spine (ROM, tenderness, Spurling).

4. Cervical/vestibular/vision screens: Dix-Hallpike if positional vertigo; near point of convergence; accommodation testing where feasible.

DIFFERENTIAL DIAGNOSIS (TOP 5)

1. Cervicogenic headache/neck strain or whiplash-associated disorder.

2. Vestibular disorders (BPPV, vestibular neuritis) and oculomotor dysfunction.

3. Migraine/vestibular migraine; medication-overuse headache.

4. Anxiety/depression/PTSD; sleep disturbance/insomnia; autonomic dysfunction (orthostatic intolerance).

5. Intracranial injury (ICH/contusion) — consider with red flags or anticoagulation.

INVESTIGATIONS (POC/LABS/IMAGING)

1. Clinical diagnosis — routine imaging is not required unless red flags. Use decision rules for CT (e.g., Canadian CT Head Rule in adults; PECARN in

children).

2. Neurocognitive tests (computerized) and balance platforms can assist but are not diagnostic; interpret in clinical context.

3. VOMS and oculomotor screening to identify treatable vestibular/ocular subtypes; Dix-Hallpike for BPPV; orthostatic vitals if dizziness/syncope.

4. Consider sleep screening tools (Insomnia Severity Index), PHQ-9/GAD-7 for mood, and Headache Impact Test (HIT-6).

MANAGEMENT (NON-PHARM → MEDS → PROCEDURES)

A. NON-PHARMACOLOGIC (CORNERSTONES)

1. Education & reassurance: avoid complete 'cocooning'. Relative rest for 24–48 h (light activities of daily living) → then graded, symptom-limited activity.

2. Return-to-learn/work: brief accommodations (reduced workload, breaks, screen filters, extra time) with stepwise increase as tolerated.

3. Return-to-sport (if relevant): follow staged progression (symptom-limited activity → light aerobic → sport-specific → non-contact drills → full practice → game), advancing ≥24 h between stages if no significant symptom worsening.

4. Aerobic exercise therapy: prescribe daily sub-symptom threshold activity (e.g., 20–30 min brisk walk/cycle)

guided by symptoms or Buffalo Concussion Treadmill Test when available.

5. Targeted rehab: vestibular therapy for dizziness/ visual motion sensitivity; oculomotor/vision therapy for convergence/accommodation issues; cervical physio for neck-driven pain/headache.

6. Sleep hygiene: regular schedule, limit naps/caffeine late day; consider melatonin. Screen/treat mood and anxiety; brief CBT components can help.

7. Driving: avoid until attention, reaction time, and symptoms (esp. dizziness/visual) normalize; workplace safety review for hazards.

B. MEDICATIONS (SYMPTOM-TARGETED; AVOID ROUTINE OPIOIDS/BENZOS)

1. Headache: acetaminophen first-line in first 24–48 h; then consider NSAIDs if no bleeding risk. For migraine phenotype: naproxen/ibuprofen or triptan (if typical migraine, no contraindications); preventive options in PPCS include amitriptyline/nortriptyline, topiramate, or propranolol — start low, monitor effects.

2. Nausea: short course ondansetron or prochlorperazine.

3. Sleep: melatonin; short-term trazodone in selected adults if insomnia persists (avoid dependence-forming meds).

4. Mood/anxiety: SSRIs/SNRIs when persistent and impairing; combine with therapy.

5. Avoid: routine opioids, benzodiazepines, and frequent

use of analgesics that risk medication-overuse headache.

C. PROCEDURES/CLINIC TOOLS

1. Perform/arrange Epley maneuver for posterior-canal BPPV when Dix-Hallpike positive.
2. Use SCAT6/Child SCAT6 (or short checklists) for standardized symptom/balance documentation at baseline and follow-ups.
3. Buffalo Concussion Treadmill or Bike Test (if trained) to set safe exercise thresholds; otherwise use self-paced symptom-limited exertion with HR logging.

DISPOSITION (DISCHARGE/OBSERVE/TRANSFER) & RETURN PRECAUTIONS

1. Immediate ED/CT pathway: any red flags (worsening headache, repeated vomiting, seizure, focal deficit, confusion/agitation, anticoagulant use with head hit, unequal pupils, severe neck pain, worsening drowsiness).
2. Urgent specialty referral (sports med/neurology/rehab) if: symptoms persist >4 weeks (adults) or >4 weeks (children) despite active management, recurrent concussions, complicated vestibular/visual deficits, significant mood disorder, school/work failure to progress.
3. Follow-up within 1–2 weeks (earlier if high-risk or athlete).

4. Return immediately for: new neuro deficits, escalating headache, repeated vomiting, syncope, severe neck pain, confusion, or behavior change.

PEARLS & PITFALLS

1. Strict rest beyond 24–48 h can slow recovery — encourage early, graded activity.
2. Treat what you find: many "concussion" symptoms are cervicogenic, vestibular, ocular, or migraine — targeted therapy speeds recovery.
3. Limit screen time and cognitive load only briefly; re-introduce as tolerated with breaks and accommodations.
4. Beware medication-overuse headache (≥15 days/ mo of simple analgesics or ≥10 days/mo of triptans/ combination analgesics).
5. Document baseline and serial symptom scores and provide written return-to-learn/work/sport plans.

REFERENCES

1. Concussion in Sport Group. 6th International Consensus Statement on Concussion in Sport (Amsterdam 2022; published 2023, open access). bjsm.bmj.com
2. SCAT6 and Child SCAT6 tools (open access). bjsm. bmj.com
3. CDC HEADS UP — Concussion and Mild TBI resources for clinicians (public). cdc.gov/headsup

4. VA/DoD Clinical Practice Guideline for the Management of Concussion-mTBI (2021, open PDF). healthquality.va.gov

5. NICE Guideline NG232. Head injury: assessment and early management (2023+, public). nice.org.uk

6. AAFP. Current Concepts in Concussion: Initial Evaluation and Management; Return-to-Play/Work guidance (open articles). aafp.org

7. Parachute Canada. Canadian Guideline on Concussion in Sport & Return-to-School/Work (open). parachute.ca

HEADACHE — FAMILY MEDICINE OFFICE

OVERVIEW & "DON'T MISS"

1. Common primary headaches: migraine (with/without aura), tension-type headache (TTH), cluster/trigeminal autonomic cephalalgias (TACs).

2. Identify secondary causes using red flags (SNNOOP10-style): systemic symptoms (fever/weight loss/cancer/HIV), neurologic deficits, sudden thunderclap onset, new onset after age 50, pattern change/progressive, positional, precipitated by cough/valsalva/exertion, papilledema, pregnancy/puerperium, painful red eye/autonomic features, post-trauma, and new meds/toxins (e.g., CO, medication overuse).

3. DON'T MISS: subarachnoid hemorrhage (thunderclap), meningitis/encephalitis, acute angle-closure glaucoma, carbon monoxide poisoning, temporal (giant cell) arteritis ≥50 y, cerebral venous sinus thrombosis (post-partum/OCP), intracranial mass/HTN, preeclampsia/eclampsia.

HISTORY & EXAM

1. Characterize: onset/time to peak, duration, frequency,

triggers (menses, sleep loss, foods), associated symptoms (nausea/vomiting, photophobia/phonophobia, aura, focal deficits), autonomic signs (lacrimation, nasal congestion, ptosis).

2. Medication use: days/month of simple analgesics, triptans, opioids, caffeine; new meds (nitrates, PDE5i, hormonal).

3. Medical history: HTN, pregnancy, immunosuppression, cancer; recent infection or head/neck trauma.

4. Exam: vitals (incl. BP), general and neuro exam, fundoscopy for papilledema, temporal artery tenderness (≥50 y), neck stiffness (meningism); eye exam and IOP if red eye/vision changes.

DIFFERENTIAL DIAGNOSIS (TOP 5)

1. Migraine (± aura).
2. Tension-type headache (episodic/chronic).
3. Cluster headache / other TACs.
4. Medication-overuse headache (MOH).
5. Secondary: SAH, meningitis, GCA, acute angle-closure glaucoma, CO poisoning.

INVESTIGATIONS (POC/LABS/IMAGING)

1. No routine imaging for typical primary headaches with normal neuro exam.

2. Urgent neuroimaging for red flags: non-contrast head CT (for thunderclap/SAH, acute neuro deficits/trauma). If CT negative and SAH still suspected (especially >6

h after onset), pursue LP and/or CT-angiography per local protocol.

3. MRI brain for atypical/chronic progressive headaches, neurologic deficits, new-onset headache with cancer/immunosuppression, trigeminal autonomic cephalalgias with atypical features.

4. Labs as indicated: ESR/CRP (GCA) in ≥50 y with new headache/visual symptoms/jaw claudication; pregnancy test in reproductive-age; CO level if exposure suspected; consider CBC, BMP if systemic illness suspected.

MANAGEMENT (NON-PHARM → MEDS → PROCEDURES)

A. NON-PHARMACOLOGIC

1. Education: diagnosis, triggers, keeping a headache diary; regular sleep/meals, hydration, exercise; limit caffeine (<200 mg/day) and alcohol.

2. Behavioral therapies: relaxation/biofeedback, CBT, mindfulness; physical therapy for cervicogenic components; blue-light/screen hygiene.

3. Avoid medication overuse: limit simple analgesics to <15 days/month and triptans/combination analgesics to <10 days/month.

B. ACUTE TREATMENT (CHOOSE BASED ON SEVERITY, NAUSEA, COMORBIDITIES)

1. Migraine (mild–moderate): NSAIDs (ibuprofen,

naproxen) or acetaminophen at onset ± antiemetic (metoclopramide 10 mg or prochlorperazine 10 mg).

2. Migraine (moderate–severe or NSAID failure): triptan (e.g., sumatriptan 50–100 mg PO or 6 mg SC; rizatriptan 10 mg; zolmitriptan 5 mg PO/NS) — avoid with significant vascular disease/uncontrolled HTN/ basilar-type aura. Consider non-oral (NS/SC) if rapid onset with vomiting.

3. Alternatives if triptans contraindicated/not tolerated: gepants (ubrogepant, rimegepant) or ditan (lasmiditan) per local availability/label.

4. Tension-type: NSAIDs/acetaminophen; avoid opioids and butalbital combos.

5. Cluster headache: high-flow oxygen via non-rebreather 12–15 L/min for 15–20 min; subcutaneous sumatriptan 6 mg or intranasal zolmitriptan; avoid oral triptans for acute cluster (onset too slow).

6. Avoid routine opioids and benzodiazepines for primary headaches.

C. PREVENTIVE TREATMENT (CONSIDER IF ≥4 MIGRAINE DAYS/MONTH, DISABLING ATTACKS, MOH, OR PATIENT PREFERENCE)

1. First-line oral options: topiramate (titrate to 50–100 mg/day), propranolol (80–160 mg/day), metoprolol, amitriptyline (10–50 mg qHS), nortriptyline, candesartan (16–32 mg/day).

2. CGRP-pathway therapies: monoclonal antibodies (erenumab, fremanezumab, galcanezumab,

eptinezumab) for episodic/chronic migraine after failure/intolerance to orals; check coverage and contraindications.

3. Chronic migraine (≥15 headache days/month): onabotulinumtoxinA 155–195 units q12 weeks (specialist).

4. Cluster prevention: verapamil (ECG monitoring for heart block), short steroid bridge at start of cluster under specialist guidance; consider lithium if refractory (monitor levels/thyroid/renal).

5. TTH prevention: amitriptyline first-line; address cervical myofascial factors.

D. SPECIAL POPULATIONS & PEARLS

1. Pregnancy/post-partum: acetaminophen first-line; metoclopramide safe; avoid NSAIDs in 3rd trimester; avoid ergot derivatives; many guidelines allow sumatriptan if benefits outweigh risks — confirm with obstetrics. New/worst headache in pregnancy/ puerperium → rule out preeclampsia/eclampsia and CVST.

2. Giant cell arteritis (≥50 y): start high-dose prednisone (e.g., 40–60 mg/day) urgently if suspected; add aspirin unless contraindicated; arrange temporal artery biopsy within ~1–2 weeks; urgent ophthalmology if visual symptoms.

3. Medication-overuse headache: educate; wean/stop overused agent (abrupt for simple analgesics/triptans; taper for opioids/barbiturates/benzodiazepines with

supports). Start/optimize prevention and bridge with NSAIDs/antiemetics/relaxation.

4. Thunderclap headache: treat as SAH until excluded — ED pathway for CT ± LP/CTA.

5. CO poisoning: consider in cluster-like headache with multiple household members symptomatic; give 100% oxygen and arrange ED evaluation.

DISPOSITION (DISCHARGE/OBSERVE/ TRANSFER) & RETURN PRECAUTIONS

1. Immediate ED/transfer: thunderclap onset, persistent neuro deficits, meningism with fever, papilledema with focal signs, acute angle-closure (red painful eye, halos, mid-dilated pupil), hypertensive emergency, pregnancy-related severe headache, suspected CO exposure.

2. Urgent (days) referral: suspected GCA, new daily persistent headache with systemic signs, refractory or atypical headaches, frequent disabling migraine despite optimized therapy.

3. Return immediately for: worsening or new neurologic symptoms, new pattern change, intractable vomiting, syncope, or chest pain with triptan use.

PEARLS & PITFALLS

1. Treat early and adequately — under-dosing acute therapy increases recurrence and MOH risk.

2. Use non-oral routes for severe nausea/vomiting and

for cluster attacks.

3. Avoid opioids and butalbital products in primary headaches.

4. Check BP, fundi, and perform focused neuro exam on all first or worst headaches.

5. Start a simple prevention when attacks are frequent or disabling; reassess monthly and step down after sustained control.

REFERENCES

1. NICE Guideline NG150. Headaches in over 12s: diagnosis and management (public). nice.org.uk

2. American Headache Society (AHS). Consensus statements and toolkits on acute and preventive migraine treatment (open resources). americanheadachesociety.org

3. AAFP. Acute Migraine Headache: Treatment Strategies; Tension-Type Headache; Cluster Headache; Giant Cell Arteritis; Subarachnoid Hemorrhage (open articles). aafp.org

4. BMJ / BASH public resources: Headache evaluation and red flags; Cluster headache and TACs (public pages). bmj.com / bash.org.uk

5. Emergency Care BC. Thunderclap Headache; Subarachnoid Hemorrhage; Acute Angle-Closure Glaucoma summaries (public). emergencycarebc.ca

6. CDC. Carbon Monoxide Poisoning — Clinical Guidance (public). cdc.gov

7. AAN patient summaries & Choosing Wisely (don't image uncomplicated headache) (public). aan.com / choosingwisely.org

MUSCULOSKELETAL & RHEUMATOLOGY

BACK PAIN — FAMILY MEDICINE OFFICE

OVERVIEW & "DON'T MISS"

1. Most back pain is non-specific and self-limited within 4–6 weeks. Identify red flags requiring urgent imaging or referral.

2. Common patterns: non-specific mechanical pain; radiculopathy (sciatica); spinal stenosis (neurogenic claudication); vertebral compression fracture; inflammatory back pain.

3. DON'T MISS: cauda equina syndrome (urinary retention/incontinence, saddle anesthesia, bilateral weakness), spinal epidural abscess/osteomyelitis (fever, IV drug use, recent infection/procedure), malignancy/metastasis (unexplained weight loss, night pain, cancer history), abdominal aortic aneurysm, renal colic, high-energy trauma/fracture.

HISTORY & EXAM

1. Onset and course: acute (<6 wks), subacute (6–12 wks), chronic (>12 wks); mechanism/trauma; night/ rest pain; radiation below knee; numbness/weakness; bowel/bladder symptoms; fever/chills; weight loss;

cancer/infection/steroid use/osteoporosis.

2. Function: effect on work/ADLs/sleep; psychosocial factors (yellow flags): mood, fear-avoidance, catastrophizing; screen for depression (PHQ-2/9).

3. Exam: vitals; inspection for deformity; palpation for midline tenderness; ROM; straight-leg raise (L5/S1), crossed SLR; femoral stretch (L2–4); full neuro (power, sensation, reflexes incl. ankle jerk), gait, heel/toe walk; consider abdominal/rectal exam if red flags (tone/perianal sensation).

DIFFERENTIAL DIAGNOSIS (TOP 5)

1. Non-specific mechanical low back pain (strain/facet/myofascial).

2. Radiculopathy from lumbar disc herniation (L4–S1).

3. Spinal stenosis (neurogenic claudication, better flexed/with shopping cart).

4. Vertebral compression fracture (age, steroids, osteoporosis).

5. Serious causes: malignancy, infection (SEA/discitis), fracture, AAA/renal colic/pancreatitis (referred).

INVESTIGATIONS (POC/LABS/IMAGING)

1. No routine imaging for acute <6 wks without red flags. Reassess in 2–4 wks.

2. Immediate imaging (ED/urgent) if: severe/progressive neuro deficits, suspected cauda equina, infection, malignancy, fracture after trauma, or AAA; MRI is

preferred for neuro/infection/malignancy; CT for fracture if MRI unavailable.

3. Consider imaging if persistent disabling radicular pain >6 wks despite guideline-directed care and considering surgery/intervention.

4. Labs when infection/malignancy suspected: CBC, ESR/CRP; blood cultures if febrile or SEA suspected; urinalysis if renal colic/UTI concerns.

5. Bone density assessment (DXA) if fragility fracture suspected or risk high.

MANAGEMENT (NON-PHARM → MEDS → PROCEDURES)

A. NON-PHARMACOLOGIC (FIRST-LINE FOR MOST)

1. Education: favorable prognosis; stay active and return to normal activity as tolerated; avoid bed rest.

2. Heat therapy; spinal manipulation/mobilization by trained provider; massage; acupuncture; structured exercise (core stabilization, McKenzie-type, walking).

3. Cognitive-behavioral strategies and address psychosocial 'yellow flags'; workplace modifications if needed.

B. MEDICATIONS (SHORTEST EFFECTIVE DURATION; REVIEW RISKS)

1. Non-specific acute pain: NSAIDs if not contraindicated;

acetaminophen has limited benefit alone but reasonable adjunct.

2. Short course skeletal muscle relaxant (e.g., cyclobenzaprine at night) can help acute severe spasm; avoid in older adults or if sedation risks.

3. Radicular pain: short course NSAIDs; consider a brief oral steroid taper only case-by-case (mixed evidence); neuropathic agents (gabapentin/duloxetine) may help chronic radicular pain — trial with monitoring.

4. Avoid routine opioids; reserve for severe acute pain unresponsive to other therapy for a few days only, with clear stop plan. Avoid benzodiazepines.

5. Topicals: NSAID gel for focal pain; lidocaine patches for myofascial pain (limited evidence).

C. PROCEDURES/REFERRALS

1. Urgent ED/neurosurgery for red flags/cauda equina, rapidly progressive deficits, severe intractable pain with systemic features.

2. Consider epidural steroid injection for persistent, function-limiting radicular pain with imaging-confirmed nerve root compression after conservative therapy (usually ≥6 weeks).

3. Refer to physiatry/physiotherapy for guided exercise; multidisciplinary pain programs for chronic disabling pain; surgical opinion for refractory neuro deficits or intolerable radiculopathy with concordant imaging.

DISPOSITION (DISCHARGE/OBSERVE/ TRANSFER) & RETURN PRECAUTIONS

1. Immediate ED/transfer: new urinary retention/ incontinence, saddle anesthesia, bilateral or rapidly progressive leg weakness; fever with severe back pain (especially IV drug use/recent skin/urinary infection); severe trauma; suspected AAA; uncontrolled pain with systemic signs.

2. Routine outpatient: most mechanical pain; follow up in 2–4 weeks to reassess pain/function and wean meds; earlier if worsening.

3. Return immediately for: new neurologic deficits, fever/ chills, severe night/rest pain, unintended weight loss, or no improvement after 4–6 weeks.

PEARLS & PITFALLS

1. No imaging in the first 6 weeks for uncomplicated low back pain — it rarely changes management.

2. Ask about cancer history, fever/IVDU, recent infection/ procedure, trauma, steroids/osteoporosis — these drive imaging and referral.

3. Radiculopathy often improves within 6–12 weeks; encourage activity and structured PT.

4. Consider shingles prodrome (back pain before rash) in neuropathic, dermatomal pain.

5. Screen and treat depression/anxiety and sleep problems — they affect outcomes.

REFERENCES

1.	NICE Guideline NG59. Low back pain and sciatica in over 16s: assessment and management (public). nice. org.uk

2.	ACP (American College of Physicians) Clinical Practice Guideline (2017): Noninvasive treatments for acute, subacute, and chronic low back pain (open access). acpjournals.org

3.	AAFP. Mechanical Low Back Pain; Choosing Wisely: Imaging for Low Back Pain; Evaluation of Low Back Pain in Adults (open articles). aafp.org

4.	CDC. 2022 Clinical Practice Guideline for Prescribing Opioids for Pain — summary (public). cdc.gov

5.	BMJ Best Practice (public summaries) & WHO resources on musculoskeletal pain and activity (public). bmj.com / who.int

6.	Emergency Care BC. Cauda Equina Syndrome; Spinal Epidural Abscess clinical summaries (public). emergencycarebc.ca

JOINT PAIN — FAMILY MEDICINE OFFICE (ARTHRALGIA/ARTHRITIS)

OVERVIEW & "DON'T MISS"

1. Differentiate inflammatory vs non-inflammatory and mono- vs oligo- vs poly-articular patterns; onset (acute <2 wks vs chronic).

2. DON'T MISS: septic arthritis (hot, swollen, very painful joint ± fever), crystalline arthritis with severe inflammation, hemarthrosis (anticoagulation/trauma), acute rheumatic fever (rare, post-strep), Lyme arthritis (endemic areas), fracture/dislocation, necrotizing infection, endocarditis related arthropathy.

HISTORY & EXAM

1. Inflammatory features: morning stiffness ≥30–60 min, improves with activity, night pain, swelling/warmth; non-inflammatory: brief stiffness, worse with use.

2. Pattern clues:

3. Acute monoarthritis → septic, gout/CPPD, hemarthrosis, trauma.

4. Oligoarthritis (≤4 joints) → reactive arthritis, Lyme,

psoriatic/enteropathic arthritis.

5. Symmetric small-joint polyarthritis → rheumatoid arthritis (RA), viral (parvo), SLE.

6. Systemic: fever, weight loss, rash (psoriasis/malar), uveitis, urethritis/cervicitis/diarrhea (reactive), tick exposure (Lyme), travel/infection, IVDU.

7. Meds: diuretics (gout), fluoroquinolones (tendinopathy), isoniazid (lupus-like), hydralazine/ minocycline/PTU (drug-induced ANCA-vasculitis).

8. Exam: map tender/swollen joints; range of motion; effusion vs periarticular pain (bursitis/tendinopathy); enthesitis/dactylitis; axial back pain tests; skin/nails, oral ulcers; heart/lungs; neurovascular status.

DIFFERENTIAL DIAGNOSIS (TOP 5)

1. Septic arthritis; crystalline arthritis (gout/CPPD); osteoarthritis; rheumatoid arthritis; spondyloarthritis (psoriatic/reactive/axial).

INVESTIGATIONS (POC/LABS/IMAGING)

1. Acute hot swollen joint → URGENT arthrocentesis BEFORE antibiotics if feasible: cell count with differential, Gram stain/culture, and crystals (polarized microscopy).

2. Basic labs (tailor): CBC, ESR/CRP; BMP/urate if gout suspected; blood cultures if septic arthritis suspected; ASO if acute rheumatic fever suspected.

3. Targeted serology only with suggestive features: RF/

anti-CCP for RA; ANA (IFA) with reflex ENA/dsDNA/ complements for CTD; HLA-B27 for spondyloarthritis context; Lyme two-tier testing in endemic exposure with compatible arthritis.

4. Imaging: X-ray for trauma/degeneration/CPPD calcifications; point-of-care ultrasound (if available) to confirm effusion/guide aspiration; MRI for occult osteomyelitis/AVN or persistent monoarthritis when indicated.

MANAGEMENT (NON-PHARM → MEDS → PROCEDURES)

A. NON-PHARMACOLOGIC

1. Rest acutely inflamed joint with brief immobilization then gradual mobilization; ice for acute, heat for chronic stiffness.

2. Weight management; exercise therapy (ROM → strengthening → aerobic); joint protection, shoe orthotics/braces as indicated; physio referral.

3. Patient education and self-management; smoking cessation (improves RA/SpA outcomes).

B. MEDICATIONS (EXAMPLES; TAILOR TO ETIOLOGY & COMORBIDITIES)

1. Septic arthritis: ED/admit for IV antibiotics and urgent orthopedics; obtain synovial and blood cultures. Avoid intra-articular steroids.

2. Gout flare: NSAIDs at anti-inflammatory doses (if no

contraindications), or low-dose colchicine (1.2 mg then 0.6 mg 1 h later; then 0.6 mg once or twice daily), or oral/IA glucocorticoids; avoid starting/stopping urate-lowering therapy during acute flare.

3. CPPD flare: NSAIDs, colchicine, or intra-articular steroids; evaluate for triggers (hyperparathyroidism, hemochromatosis).

4. Osteoarthritis: topical NSAIDs (knee/hand) first-line; oral NSAIDs if needed/low risk; acetaminophen modest; duloxetine for chronic knee OA pain; intra-articular corticosteroid short-term relief; avoid chronic opioids.

5. RA/suspected inflammatory polyarthritis: early rheumatology referral for DMARDs; short NSAIDs for symptom relief; avoid prolonged steroids — brief low-dose prednisone only as bridge when necessary.

6. Reactive arthritis: treat inciting infection (e.g., doxycycline for Chlamydia per guidelines); NSAIDs; short steroids for severe synovitis; ophthalmology for uveitis.

7. Bursitis/tendinopathy: activity modification, physio, topical NSAIDs; consider ultrasound-guided steroid injection for persistent cases (after excluding infection).

C. PROCEDURES

1. Arthrocentesis for diagnostic clarity in monoarthritis; therapeutic aspiration + intra-articular steroid for non-infectious inflammatory effusions.

2. Joint injections should be sterile technique; defer

steroids if infection not excluded; counsel on rest 24–48 h post-injection.

DISPOSITION (DISCHARGE/OBSERVE/ TRANSFER) & RETURN PRECAUTIONS

1. Immediate ED/orthopedics: suspected septic arthritis (fever, inability to bear weight, severe pain, high CRP), rapidly progressive neurologic deficits, fracture/dislocation, hemarthrosis with anticoagulation instability.

2. Urgent (days) rheumatology: new inflammatory polyarthritis (>6 wks), recurrent hot monoarthritis, positive anti-CCP/ANA with organ features, persistent monoarthritis despite negative initial work-up.

3. Return immediately for: fever, rapidly worsening swelling/redness, severe pain unresponsive to meds, new joint locking/giving way.

PEARLS & PITFALLS

1. A hot joint is septic until proven otherwise — aspirate if feasible before antibiotics.

2. Serum urate can be normal during an acute gout flare; crystals in synovial fluid are diagnostic.

3. Don't shotgun autoantibody panels — order targeted tests driven by clinical phenotype.

4. Consider crystalline disease and infection even in established RA/OA when a single joint acutely worsens.

5. Check for red flags (fever, weight loss, night pain, IVDU, immunosuppression) and reassess early if course deviates.

REFERENCES

1. NICE CKS. Gout; Septic arthritis; Rheumatoid arthritis; Spondyloarthritis; Osteoarthritis — assessment/ management (public). cks.nice.org.uk

2. AAFP. Acute Monoarthritis: Diagnosis in Adults; Gout: Rapid Evidence Review; Septic Arthritis: Diagnosis and Treatment; Osteoarthritis: Rapid Evidence Review (open). aafp.org

3. EULAR/ACR public summaries & patient resources for RA, gout, CPPD, spondyloarthritis (open). eular.org / rheumatology.org

4. Emergency Care BC. Septic Arthritis clinical summary (public). emergencycarebc.ca

5. CDC. Lyme disease — clinical care and arthritis (public). cdc.gov

6. ARUP Consult. Rheumatologic tests overview (ANA, RF, anti-CCP) — when to order, interpretation (open). arupconsult.com

7. NIH MedlinePlus. Joint pain; Osteoarthritis; Rheumatoid arthritis; Gout (public). medlineplus.gov

ARTHRITIS — RHEUMATOLOGIC & OTHER AUTOIMMUNE

OVERVIEW & "DON'T MISS"

1. Arthritis can be mechanical (OA), inflammatory (RA, psoriatic arthritis, axial/peripheral spondyloarthritis), crystalline (gout/CPPD), infectious (septic), or part of systemic autoimmune disease (SLE, vasculitis).

2. Inflammatory arthritis: morning stiffness ≥30–60 min, improves with activity; swelling, warmth, prolonged gelling. Mechanical: brief stiffness, worse with use.

3. DON'T MISS: septic arthritis (hot, swollen, very painful single joint + fever) → urgent ED/aspiration/ IV antibiotics; acute back pain with neurologic deficits (cauda equina); rapidly evolving weakness or systemic symptoms (SLE/vasculitis flare); ocular inflammation (uveitis) in spondyloarthritis.

HISTORY & EXAM

1. Pattern: number of joints (mono/oligo/poly), symmetry, small vs large joints, axial involvement, onset/duration, flares.

2. Extra-articular: psoriasis/skin/nails; IBD/diarrhea; uveitis; dactylitis/enthesitis; oral/nasal ulcers; photosensitive rash; Raynaud; sicca; fevers/weight loss.

3. Precipitants: trauma, infection (post-streptococcal/ reactive), new meds (diuretics for gout), alcohol. Family history (psoriasis, spondyloarthritis, gout).

4. Exam: joint swelling/tenderness/ROM; pattern (MCP/ PIP/MTP in RA; DIP/enthesitis/dactylitis in PsA); spinal mobility (Schober) and SI joint tenderness; tophi; nail pitting; rash; oral ulcers; eye redness/photophobia.

DIFFERENTIAL DIAGNOSIS (TOP 5)

1. Rheumatoid arthritis (RA) — chronic symmetric small-joint inflammatory polyarthritis (≥6 wks).

2. Spondyloarthritis (axial, peripheral, psoriatic, reactive, IBD-associated).

3. Crystal arthropathies — gout (urate) and CPPD (pseudogout).

4. Osteoarthritis (OA) — mechanical pain, brief stiffness, bony enlargement.

5. Septic arthritis — especially if monoarthritis, fever, immunosuppressed, or prosthetic joint.

INVESTIGATIONS (POC/LABS/IMAGING)

1. If hot, swollen monoarthritis → URGENT arthrocentesis: Gram stain/culture, WBC count, and crystals (polarized microscopy). Treat as septic until

proven otherwise.

2. Inflammatory markers: ESR/CRP (supportive, not diagnostic). CBC, CMP (baseline for meds). Uric acid (not diagnostic during acute flare).

3. RA: RF and anti-CCP (anti-CCP is more specific); baseline hand/foot X-rays if persistent symptoms.

4. Spondyloarthritis: HLA-B27 (supportive), pelvis X-ray for sacroiliitis; consider MRI SI joints if early disease.

5. SLE/CTD when clinically suspected: ANA (screen), with reflex ENA/dsDNA/complements/urinalysis if ANA positive and features consistent; avoid indiscriminate ANA ordering.

6. Imaging: ultrasound can detect synovitis/effusions and guide injections; X-rays for erosions (RA), joint space narrowing/osteophytes (OA), chondrocalcinosis (CPPD).

7. Pre-DMARD screen (if likely): TB (IGRA/TST), Hep B/C, HIV; vaccines update (see below).

MANAGEMENT (NON-PHARM → MEDS → PROCEDURES)

A. NON-PHARMACOLOGIC

1. Education: disease course, flare management, joint protection, pacing; smoking cessation (key in RA/SpA), weight loss for OA/gout.

2. Exercise/physio: range-of-motion, strengthening, aerobic exercise; splints for RA hand/wrist; footwear/

orthotics for foot arthritis.

3. Vaccines before immunosuppression: influenza, COVID-19, pneumococcal, zoster (recombinant), Hep B; avoid live vaccines once on significant immunosuppression.

4. Comorbidity care: CV risk in RA/psoriasis, bone health (steroids), mood, sleep, work/ADLs.

B. MEDICATIONS (EXAMPLES; TAILOR TO DIAGNOSIS; CONFIRM LABS/ CONTRAINDICATIONS)

1. Symptom control: topical NSAIDs for OA hands/knees; oral NSAIDs or COX-2 if low GI/CV risk; PPI protection in high-risk; avoid in CKD/ulcer/CVD; consider acetaminophen; short oral steroids only as bridge for inflammatory disease if needed.

2. RA (suspected >6 wks): early rheumatology referral for treat-to-target. First-line csDMARD: methotrexate (once weekly) + folic acid; monitor CBC/LFT/Cr; contraindicated in pregnancy/liver disease/alcohol misuse. Alternatives/intolerance: leflunomide, sulfasalazine, hydroxychloroquine. Short course low-dose prednisone as bridge if needed.

3. Psoriatic/peripheral SpA: NSAIDs first; csDMARDs (methotrexate, sulfasalazine) for peripheral disease. Enthesitis/axial disease often needs biologics (TNF-α or IL-17 inhibitors) — specialist-led.

4. Axial spondyloarthritis: NSAIDs, physio; biologic therapy if persistent high activity — rheumatology.

5. Gout: acute flare — NSAID, colchicine (1.2 mg then 0.6 mg 1 h later, then 0.6 mg once/twice daily), or oral steroids; ice and rest. Start urate-lowering therapy (ULT) for recurrent flares/tophi/CKD/urate stones: allopurinol first-line, start low (e.g., 100 mg/day; 50 mg/day in CKD) and titrate to target serum urate <360 μmol/L (<6 mg/dL); prophylaxis with low-dose colchicine or NSAID during ULT initiation. Consider HLA-B*58:01 testing in high-risk ancestry (e.g., Han Chinese, Thai, Korean with CKD).

6. CPPD: acute — NSAIDs/colchicine/steroids; search for triggers (hyperparathyroidism, hemochromatosis).

7. SLE: hydroxychloroquine is foundational (baseline/annual eye exams); steroids/sparing agents by specialist.

8. Intra-articular corticosteroid injections: effective for single-joint flares (OA/RA/CPPD) — ensure no sepsis first.

C. PROCEDURES

1. Joint aspiration/injection (aseptic technique) for diagnosis and symptom control; send fluid for crystal/Gram/culture.

2. Order and interpret screening labs before DMARD/biologic therapy; coordinate vaccine updates prior to initiation.

DISPOSITION (DISCHARGE/OBSERVE/ TRANSFER) & RETURN PRECAUTIONS

1. Refer to rheumatology: suspected new inflammatory arthritis >6 weeks, axial symptoms with inflammatory back pain, persistent enthesitis/dactylitis, recurrent gout with tophi, suspected SLE/vasculitis, abnormal imaging suggestive of erosive disease.

2. ED/urgent same-day: suspected septic arthritis, rapidly progressive neurologic deficits, severe ocular inflammation (uveitis), febrile neutropenia on immunosuppression, uncontrolled pain/swelling with fever.

3. Return urgently for: fever on DMARD/biologic, new chest pain/SOB, hematuria/foamy urine (SLE), vision changes, or severe flare not improving within 48–72 h of treatment.

PEARLS & PITFALLS

1. Don't rely on uric acid during an acute gout flare — it may be normal; diagnosis is clinical ± crystal proof.

2. Order ANA only when clinical features suggest CTD; a positive ANA alone is nonspecific.

3. Anti-CCP supports RA diagnosis and predicts erosive disease; start DMARDs early via rheumatology.

4. Screen for TB/Hep B/C before biologics; update vaccines first (avoid live vaccines on significant immunosuppression).

5. Smoking cessation improves RA/SpA outcomes and

reduces CV risk.

REFERENCES

1. NICE Guideline NG100. Rheumatoid arthritis in adults: management; and CKS: Rheumatoid arthritis (public). nice.org.uk / cks.nice.org.uk

2. NICE Guideline NG65. Spondyloarthritis in over 16s (axial & peripheral, including psoriatic arthritis) (public). nice.org.uk

3. NICE Guideline NG219. Gout: diagnosis and management (public). nice.org.uk

4. NICE Guideline NG226. Osteoarthritis in over 16s: diagnosis and management (public). nice.org.uk

5. AAFP. Diagnosis and Management of Rheumatoid Arthritis; Gout: Rapid Evidence Review; Septic Arthritis: Diagnosis and Treatment (open articles). aafp.org

6. Emergency Care BC. Septic Arthritis — Clinical Summary (public). emergencycarebc.ca

7. EULAR/ACR public summaries & patient resources on RA/PsA/axSpA/SLE (open pages). eular.org / rheumatology.org

8. Choosing Wisely Canada. Rheumatology recommendations (ANA/RF ordering, imaging) (public). choosingwiselycanada.org

DIAGNOSIS OF RHEUMATOLOGIC & AUTOIMMUNE DISEASE

OVERVIEW & "DON'T MISS"

1. Diagnosis hinges on PATTERN RECOGNITION (joint distribution, systemic features) + TARGETED tests. Avoid indiscriminate 'autoimmune panels'.

2. Inflammatory arthritis → morning stiffness ≥30–60 min, improves with activity; mechanical pain → worse with use, brief stiffness.

3. DON'T MISS: septic arthritis; giant cell arteritis with visual symptoms; pulmonary-renal vasculitis (hemoptysis + hematuria/RBC casts); scleroderma renal crisis (abrupt HTN + AKI); severe uveitis; catastrophic APS.

HISTORY & EXAM

1. Pattern: mono/oligo/poly; symmetric vs asymmetric; small vs large joints; axial involvement; enthesitis/ dactylitis; rashes (malar/photosensitive, psoriasis), oral/nasal ulcers; Raynaud; sicca (dry eyes/mouth); serositis; neuro/psych; fevers/weight loss.

2. Triggers/risks: infections, medications (hydralazine, minocycline, procainamide, TNF-inhibitors), cocaine/ levamisole, smoking (RA/SpA), family history (psoriasis/IBD/SpA).

3. Exam: swollen/tender joints; nail pitting; tophi; oral ulcers; photosensitive rash; livedo/purpura; sclerodactyly/telangiectasias; parotid enlargement; lung crackles; BP; eye redness/photophobia; neuro screen.

DIFFERENTIAL DIAGNOSIS (TOP 5)

1. Inflammatory arthritis: rheumatoid arthritis; spondyloarthritis (axial/peripheral/psoriatic/reactive/ IBD-related).

2. Connective-tissue disease (CTD): SLE, Sjögren, systemic sclerosis, inflammatory myopathies, MCTD.

3. Vasculitides: ANCA-associated (GPA/MPA), IgA vasculitis, PAN; anti-GBM disease.

4. Crystal arthropathies: gout/CPPD (pseudogout).

5. Mimics: infections (parvovirus, hepatitis B/C, endocarditis, TB), malignancy (lymphoma), endocrine (thyroid), drug-induced syndromes.

INVESTIGATIONS (POC/LABS/IMAGING)

1. Baseline for most suspected inflammatory disease: CBC (cytopenias), CMP (Cr/LFTs), ESR/CRP, urinalysis with microscopy (protein/hematuria/RBC casts).

2. Rheumatoid arthritis suspected (≥6 wks symmetric small-joint swelling): RF and anti-CCP (anti-CCP more specific); hand/foot X-rays baseline; MSK ultrasound can detect synovitis/erosions.

3. Spondyloarthritis suspected (inflammatory back pain, enthesitis, dactylitis, uveitis/psoriasis/IBD): CRP; HLA-B27 (supportive, not diagnostic); pelvis X-ray (sacroiliitis) or MRI SI joints in early disease.

4. SLE/CTD suspected (pattern-based): order ANA (IFA method preferred). If ANA positive with compatible features → reflex tests: dsDNA, ENA (Sm/RNP/ SSA/SSB), complements (C3/C4), direct Coombs as indicated; repeat UA and protein:Cr ratio.

5. Sjögren suspected: SSA/SSB; objective sicca tests (Schirmer, ocular staining); consider salivary gland US/ biopsy via specialist.

6. Systemic sclerosis suspected: ANA pattern (centromere vs nucleolar), anticentromere/Scl-70/RNA polymerase III; nailfold capillaroscopy; screen for ILD (PFTs ± HRCT) and pulmonary hypertension (echo).

7. Myositis suspected: CK, aldolase, AST/ALT, LDH; myositis-specific antibodies (e.g., anti-Jo-1, Mi-2, SRP, MDA5) if available; EMG/MRI muscle and consider biopsy via specialist.

8. Vasculitis suspected: urinalysis (RBC casts), renal function; ANCA (PR3/MPO) ONLY if clinical features suggest AAV (ENT/lung/kidney, palpable purpura, neuropathy); consider anti-GBM if pulmonary-renal; obtain tissue biopsy when feasible (temporal artery,

kidney, skin).

9. Crystal disease: arthrocentesis for polarized microscopy is gold standard; serum uric acid not diagnostic during acute gout flare; CPPD shows chondrocalcinosis on X-ray.

10. Infection/malignancy screens as guided: hepatitis B/C, HIV, TB testing; blood cultures if endocarditis suspected; CXR for sarcoid/vasculitis; SPEP if myeloma concern.

MANAGEMENT (NON-PHARM → MEDS → PROCEDURES)

A. NON-PHARMACOLOGIC (DIAGNOSTIC PHASE)

1. Education: explain that many autoantibodies are supportive, not diagnostic; diagnosis integrates clinical pattern + labs + imaging + sometimes biopsy.

2. Lifestyle: smoking cessation (improves RA/SpA outcomes), exercise and joint protection; sun protection in suspected cutaneous lupus.

3. Vaccines: update influenza, COVID-19, pneumococcal, and zoster before immunosuppression; avoid live vaccines once on significant immunosuppression.

B. MEDICATIONS (WHILE CLARIFYING DIAGNOSIS)

1. Symptom relief: topical NSAIDs for OA-type pain; NSAIDs/COX-2 cautiously for inflammatory symptoms if renal/GI/CV risk acceptable; PPI prophylaxis in

high-risk.

2. Short prednisone tapers can cloud diagnosis (and precipitate scleroderma renal crisis); avoid unless urgent indications (e.g., GCA, severe organ-threatening disease) — then involve specialists.

3. If persistent inflammatory arthritis (>6 wks) strongly suggests RA/SpA → expedite rheumatology for early DMARD/biologic initiation; avoid prolonged steroids/ NSAID monotherapy.

C. PROCEDURES

1. Arthrocentesis for any undifferentiated acutely swollen joint — send cell count with differential, Gram stain/ culture, and crystals.

2. Coordinate tissue biopsy when indicated: temporal artery (GCA), kidney/skin/nerve (vasculitis), salivary gland (Sjögren), muscle (myositis).

3. Use MSK ultrasound (if trained/access) to detect synovitis, power Doppler activity, and guide aspiration/ injection.

DISPOSITION (DISCHARGE/OBSERVE/ TRANSFER) & RETURN PRECAUTIONS

1. Immediate ED/transfer: suspected septic arthritis; visual symptoms in possible GCA; pulmonary hemorrhage; rapidly progressive GN (oliguria, RBC casts, creatinine rise); severe uveitis with vision drop; severe myositis with dysphagia/respiratory weakness.

2. Urgent (days) rheumatology/nephrology/ophthalmology: new inflammatory arthritis >6 wks; positive ANA with renal/hematologic or CNS features; ANCA-positive with systemic features; suspected myositis with CK elevation; suspected systemic sclerosis with new HTN/AKI or ILD signs.

3. Return immediately for: fever, new chest pain/SOB, hematuria/foamy urine, vision change, focal neurologic deficits, severe uncontrolled pain/swelling.

PEARLS & PITFALLS

1. Order ANA only when specific features suggest CTD — a positive ANA alone is common in healthy people and rises with age.

2. Use ANA by IFA where possible; if positive, interpret titer/pattern and test reflex antibodies guided by the clinical picture — don't shotgun ENA/dsDNA without indication.

3. Anti-CCP is more specific than RF for RA and predicts erosive disease; HLA-B27 supports but does not confirm SpA; ANCA is helpful only with the right clinical context.

4. Always check urinalysis when CTD or vasculitis is suspected — early nephritis can be silent.

5. Think infections (HBV/HCV/HIV, TB, parvovirus) and malignancy mimics before labeling 'autoimmune'. Treat the patient, not the lab result.

REFERENCES

1. NICE CKS. Rheumatoid arthritis; Spondyloarthritis; Systemic lupus erythematosus; Sjögren's; Giant cell arteritis; Vasculitis — assessment and testing (public). cks.nice.org.uk

2. AAFP. Diagnostic Approach to Polyarticular Joint Pain; Acute Monoarthritis; Rheumatologic Tests: A Primer for Family Physicians; The ANA Test — When to Order, How to Interpret (open articles). aafp.org

3. EULAR & ACR public resources and patient/clinician summaries for RA/SLE/SpA/Sjögren/Systemic Sclerosis/Myositis (open). eular.org / rheumatology.org

4. ARUP Consult — Autoimmune laboratory testing guidance: ANA by IFA, Anti-CCP, ANCA, ENA panels (open). arupconsult.com

5. Emergency Care BC. Septic Arthritis; Temporal Arteritis; Vasculitis clinical summaries (public). emergencycarebc.ca

6. Choosing Wisely (US/Canada). Recommendations on ANA/autoantibody testing and imaging in rheumatology (public). choosingwisely.org / choosingwiselycanada.org

DO NOT MISS RHEUMATOLOGIC DISORDERS — RED FLAGS IN THE FAMILY OFFICE

OVERVIEW & "DON'T MISS"

1. Recognize organ- or life-threatening rheumatologic presentations that need immediate action + referral.

2. Top emergencies to never miss:

3. Septic arthritis (hot, swollen joint with fever or severe pain).

4. Giant cell arteritis (new headache, jaw claudication, scalp tenderness, vision symptoms) — risk of blindness.

5. Pulmonary-renal vasculitis (ANCA-associated) — hemoptysis, dyspnea, rapidly rising creatinine, RBC casts.

6. SLE flare with nephritis or cerebritis — edema, hematuria/proteinuria, seizures/psychosis.

7. Scleroderma renal crisis — abrupt severe hypertension, AKI, microangiopathic hemolysis.

8. Acute inflammatory myopathy with respiratory or

bulbar involvement; or myositis-associated interstitial lung disease.

9. Catastrophic antiphospholipid syndrome (CAPS) — multiorgan thrombosis; or first unprovoked clot with classic APS features (arterial/venous thrombosis, pregnancy morbidity).

10. Sight-threatening uveitis in spondyloarthritis — painful red eye with photophobia and decreased vision.

HISTORY & EXAM

1. Timeline: acute mono- vs insidious polyarthritis; systemic symptoms (fever, weight loss, night sweats).

2. Red-flag questions: visual loss, jaw pain with chewing, hemoptysis, chest pain/SOB, hematuria/foamy urine, neuro deficits/seizures, rapidly rising BP, new clots or miscarriages.

3. Triggers/risks: recent infection/procedures, immunosuppression/steroids, pregnancy/post-partum, cocaine/levamisole, meds (hydralazine, minocycline, PTU), high-dose steroids in scleroderma.

4. Exam: vitals (especially BP), complete joint exam, temporal artery/scalp tenderness, eye exam (conjunctival injection/photophobia), lung crackles/ hemoptysis signs, edema, rashes (malar, palpable purpura, gottron papules), oral/nasal ulcers, Raynaud changes, neuro screen.

DIFFERENTIAL DIAGNOSIS (TOP 5)

1. Septic arthritis vs crystal arthritis (gout/CPPD) vs inflammatory arthritis flare.

2. GCA/large-vessel vasculitis vs tension/migraine vs TMJ disease.

3. ANCA-vasculitis vs pulmonary edema/pneumonia + AKI from other causes.

4. SLE nephritis vs diabetic/HTN nephropathy vs drug-induced lupus.

5. Scleroderma renal crisis vs malignant HTN/TMA (consider drugs, pregnancy-related).

INVESTIGATIONS (POC/LABS/IMAGING)

1. If hot, swollen joint → URGENT arthrocentesis BEFORE antibiotics if feasible: cell count with differential, Gram stain/culture, and crystals. Don't delay ED transfer if sepsis suspected.

2. GCA suspected: ESR/CRP, platelets (may be elevated), CBC; arrange SAME-DAY ophthalmology if visual symptoms; temporal artery ultrasound/biopsy — start steroids immediately (see below).

3. Pulmonary-renal/vasculitis: CBC, CMP/creatinine, urinalysis (RBC casts, protein), ANCA (PR3/MPO), C3/C4; CXR for pulmonary hemorrhage. Consider anti-GBM if pulmonary-renal with negative ANCA.

4. SLE flare: CBC, creatinine, urinalysis with microscopy, urine protein:Cr ratio, complements (C3/C4), anti-dsDNA; consider antiphospholipid panel if clotting

history.

5. Scleroderma renal crisis: BP, creatinine, urinalysis (protein/hematuria), hemolysis labs (LDH/haptoglobin/smear), renin; avoid delay in treatment.

6. Myositis: CK, aldolase, AST/ALT, LDH; if respiratory symptoms → CXR ± HRCT; review statin history and consider HMG-CoA reductase Ab if necrotizing myopathy suspected.

7. Uveitis: slit-lamp if available; otherwise urgent ophthalmology. Consider HLA-B27 in recurrent cases after acute care.

8. Order ANA and ENA panels only when clinical features suggest CTD; positive ANA alone is nonspecific.

MANAGEMENT (NON-PHARM → MEDS → PROCEDURES)

A. NON-PHARMACOLOGIC

1. Stabilize ABCs; monitor vitals and urine output if systemic illness suspected; keep NPO if procedures/transfer likely.

2. Avoid high-dose steroids in undifferentiated infection-prone presentations (e.g., hot joint) — EXCEPT start promptly for suspected GCA or life-threatening vasculitis per below.

B. MEDICATIONS (INITIAL STEPS; MANY ARE SPECIALIST-LED)

1. Septic arthritis: urgent ED/orthopedics; obtain cultures; start empiric IV antibiotics (e.g., vancomycin + third-gen cephalosporin) after aspiration if possible.

2. Giant cell arteritis: start prednisone 40–60 mg/ day immediately; if visual symptoms or neurologic ischemia, give IV methylprednisolone 500–1000 mg/ day for 3 days when possible then high-dose PO. Add low-dose aspirin if no contraindication; arrange temporal artery US/biopsy within 1–2 weeks; urgent rheumatology/ophthalmology.

3. ANCA-associated pulmonary-renal vasculitis: ED admission for pulse IV glucocorticoids and immunosuppression (rituximab/cyclophosphamide) — specialist-led; supportive care (oxygen, transfuse PRN).

4. SLE nephritis/cerebritis: ED/rheumatology for high-dose steroids ± immunosuppressants; manage hypertension and proteinuria; infection prophylaxis as indicated.

5. Scleroderma renal crisis: start ACE inhibitor immediately (captopril titrated rapidly); control BP; avoid high-dose steroids; nephrology urgent.

6. Uveitis: cycloplegic drops and URGENT ophthalmology for steroid drops/systemic therapy; exclude infections (HSV/TB) before steroids.

7. APS with acute thrombosis: anticoagulate per VTE/ arterial protocols; involve hematology/rheumatology (warfarin often used long-term).

C. PROCEDURES

1. Arthrocentesis for any undifferentiated acutely swollen joint unless prosthetic joint or overlying cellulitis — then consult.

2. Temporal artery ultrasound/biopsy arranged urgently for GCA (do not delay steroids).

3. Urine protein quantification (spot protein:creatinine) for suspected nephritis; consider renal biopsy via nephrology for glomerulonephritis.

DISPOSITION (DISCHARGE/OBSERVE/ TRANSFER) & RETURN PRECAUTIONS

1. Immediate ED/transfer: suspected septic arthritis; GCA with visual symptoms; pulmonary hemorrhage/ hemoptysis; rapidly rising creatinine with active urine sediment; severe hypertension with AKI (scleroderma); myositis with respiratory weakness; CAPS or new arterial thrombosis; severe uveitis with decreased vision.

2. Urgent (24–72 h) specialty follow-up: new inflammatory arthritis >6 weeks, recurrent uveitis without vision loss, suspected SLE without severe organ involvement, elevated complements/ autoantibodies with concerning symptoms.

3. Safety-net: written return precautions — fever, worsening pain/swelling, vision change, dyspnea/ hemoptysis, oliguria, severe headache/hypertension, neurologic symptoms.

PEARLS & PITFALLS

1. Treat GCA immediately — vision loss can be permanent; biopsy can remain positive for ~1–2 weeks after starting steroids.

2. A hot joint is septic until proven otherwise — always aspirate if feasible before antibiotics.

3. Avoid high-dose steroids in scleroderma (risk of renal crisis); if crisis occurs, ACE inhibitor is the treatment.

4. ANA positivity is common in healthy people; test only when features suggest CTD.

5. Check urine (protein/hematuria) in any suspected systemic rheumatic flare — renal involvement changes urgency.

REFERENCES

1. NICE CKS. Giant cell arteritis; Polymyalgia rheumatica; Rheumatoid arthritis; Systemic lupus erythematosus; Vasculitis (public). cks.nice.org.uk

2. AAFP. Diagnosis and Management of GCA; Acute Monoarthritis; ANCA-Associated Vasculitis; SLE: Primary Care Review (open articles). aafp.org

3. EULAR/ACR public summaries and patient resources for GCA/PMR, SLE, ANCA-vasculitis, Scleroderma, Myositis (open). eular.org / rheumatology.org

4. Emergency Care BC. Septic Arthritis; Temporal Arteritis — clinical summaries (public). emergencycarebc.ca

5. British Society for Rheumatology (BSR) guideline

summaries for GCA/PMR and ANCA vasculitis (open summaries). rheumatology.org.uk

6. Canadian Rheumatology Association & Arthritis Society Canada — patient/clinician resources (public). rheum.ca / arthritis.ca

OSTEOPOROSIS

OVERVIEW & "DON'T MISS"

1. Systemic skeletal disorder with low bone strength predisposing to fragility fractures (hip, vertebra, wrist). Common, often silent until fracture.

2. Assess fracture risk (Canada-specific FRAX ± BMD). Consider secondary causes and vertebral fractures (often occult).

3. DON'T MISS: new severe back pain with height loss/kyphosis → urgent spine X-ray/VFA for vertebral compression fracture; hip fracture after low-trauma fall → urgent ED; hypercalcemia, bone pain, anemia, renal impairment → consider myeloma/other pathology.

HISTORY & EXAM

1. History: prior fragility fracture; family history (hip fracture); falls; glucocorticoids; smoking; alcohol; low BMI; menopause age; hypogonadism; malabsorption (celiac, IBD); thyroid/parathyroid disease; kidney/liver disease; RA; meds (aromatase inhibitors, ADT, anticonvulsants, PPIs); vitamin D/calcium intake; physical activity.

2. Symptoms: back pain, height loss, dowager's hump, decreased function; red flags for malignancy/infection when pain is severe or systemic symptoms present.

3. Exam: height (current vs. peak), kyphosis, tenderness over vertebrae, gait/balance, fall risk assessment; dental issues if planning antiresorptives.

DIFFERENTIAL DIAGNOSIS (TOP 5)

1. Osteomalacia (vitamin D deficiency, low Ca/PO4, high ALP) — bone pain, proximal myopathy.

2. Multiple myeloma (bone pain, anemia, renal dysfunction, hypercalcemia).

3. Metastatic bone disease (history of cancer, focal bone pain).

4. Primary hyperparathyroidism (hypercalcemia, kidney stones, low BMD).

5. Vertebral fracture due to trauma or other causes (spondylotic changes).

INVESTIGATIONS (POC/LABS/IMAGING)

1. Risk tools: Canada-FRAX (clinical ± with BMD).

2. BMD: DXA of femoral neck (± total hip, lumbar spine) when indicated; Vertebral Fracture Assessment (VFA)/ lateral spine X-ray if age ≥65 with T-score ≤ –2.5 or FRAX 10-yr MOF 15–19.9%, or clinical suspicion.

3. Baseline labs (screen secondary causes): CBC, electrolytes/creatinine/eGFR, calcium, phosphate, albumin, ALP, AST/ALT, 25-OH vitamin D; TSH

if indicated; consider PTH, serum/urine protein electrophoresis, celiac serology (tTG-IgA), testosterone (men), cortisol (if Cushing suspected).

4. Additional: consider renal ultrasound or other imaging only if clinical suspicion of secondary cause.

MANAGEMENT (NON-PHARM → MEDS → PROCEDURES)

A. NON-PHARMACOLOGIC

1. Exercise: balance + functional training ≥2x/week; add resistance training; progress intensity safely. Avoid rapid, repetitive or end-range spinal flexion/twisting in high-risk patients.

2. Nutrition: meet Health Canada RDA — Calcium 1000 mg/day (males 51–70) and 1200 mg/day (females >50, males >70); Vitamin D RDA 600 IU/day (51–70) and 800 IU/day (>70). Adults >50 typically need a daily vitamin D supplement of 400 IU to reach RDA. Ensure adequate protein.

3. Falls prevention: home safety, vision/hearing, meds review (sedatives/antihypertensives), footwear; smoking cessation; alcohol moderation.

B. PHARMACOLOGIC (EXAMPLES; INDIVIDUALIZE TO RISK & COMORBIDITIES)

1. WHO TO TREAT (adults ≥50): prior hip/vertebral/≥2 fragility fractures; or 10-yr MOF risk ≥20%; or age ≥70 with T-score ≤ −2.5. Consider treatment if 10-yr risk

15–19.9% or <70 with T-score ≤ −2.5.

2. First-line: oral/IV bisphosphonates — e.g., alendronate 70 mg weekly; risedronate 35 mg weekly (or 150 mg monthly); zoledronic acid 5 mg IV yearly. Ensure adequate Ca/Vit D; check creatinine; counsel on rare ONJ/AFF risks.

3. Second-line / when bisphosphonates unsuitable: denosumab 60 mg SC every 6 months. IMPORTANT: do not delay or stop without a transition plan to a bisphosphonate (risk of rapid bone loss & multiple vertebral fractures).

4. Very high risk/severe vertebral fracture phenotype: consider anabolic therapy (e.g., teriparatide up to 24 months or romosozumab up to 12 months, then antiresorptive). Use specialist guidance; assess CV risk with romosozumab.

5. Drug duration/monitoring: oral bisphosphonates typically 3–6 years then consider holiday if low-to-moderate risk; no holiday for denosumab — plan sequential therapy. Monitor adherence, symptoms, Ca/Cr after IV or denosumab if at risk.

C. PROCEDURES

1. None in primary care for uncomplicated osteoporosis. Vertebral augmentation rarely and only in select cases; refer to spine specialist if intractable pain with acute vertebral compression fracture.

DISPOSITION (DISCHARGE/OBSERVE/ TRANSFER) & RETURN PRECAUTIONS

1. Discharge: most stable outpatients — initiate lifestyle/ meds as indicated; arrange follow-up in 3–6 months with adherence check and risk review.

2. Observe/urgent same-day: new moderate–severe vertebral pain without red flags, uncontrolled pain, or uncertainty about fracture → urgent imaging and analgesia plan.

3. Transfer to ED: suspected hip fracture or spinal cord compromise; red flags (fever, neuro deficits, suspected cancer, cauda equina).

4. Return immediately if: new severe back/hip pain after minor trauma; numbness/weakness; bowel/bladder symptoms; or if denosumab injection is overdue (>7 months).

PEARLS & PITFALLS

1. Don't diagnose on T-score alone — treat the PATIENT & absolute fracture risk.

2. Order VFA or lateral spine imaging when risk is borderline — occult vertebral fractures up-classify risk.

3. If using denosumab, schedule the next dose at 6 months and arrange bisphosphonate transition if stopping.

4. Check for secondary causes and fracture-promoting meds (glucocorticoids, AI, ADT, PPIs, anticonvulsants).

5. Reassess BMD based on risk: 3–10 years per

guideline; sooner if new fracture or major therapy change.

REFERENCES

1. Morin SN, Feldman S, Funnell L, et al. Clinical practice guideline for management of osteoporosis and fracture prevention in Canada: 2023 update. CMAJ. 2023;195(39):E1333–E1348. (Open access)

2. Canadian Task Force on Preventive Health Care. Fragility Fractures (2023) — Risk-assessment-first screening recommendations for females ≥65; decision aid & FRAX-Canada.

3. Osteoporosis Canada. Executive Summary — 2023 Clinical Practice Guideline (denosumab timing and duration considerations).

4. Osteoporosis Canada. 2023 Starting Medication — Bisphosphonates first-line; denosumab second-line when appropriate.

5. NICE CG146. Osteoporosis: assessing the risk of fragility fracture — selection and use of risk assessment tools (last reviewed 2024).

6. Health Canada. Vitamin D — guidance for adults including supplement of 400 IU/day for adults >50; Dietary Reference Intakes tables for Calcium & Vitamin D (2023).

7. BC Guidelines (web). Osteoporosis — Diagnosis, Treatment and Fracture Prevention (page updated 2023).

DERMATOLOGY

CONCERNING RASH IN FAMILY PRACTICE

OVERVIEW & "DON'T MISS"

1. Identify unstable patients (ABCs, vitals). Certain rashes signal life-threatening disease requiring immediate action.

2. DON'T MISS patterns:

3. Non-blanching petechiae/purpura with fever → meningococcemia, DIC, Rocky Mountain spotted fever (RMSF).

4. Pain out of proportion, rapidly spreading erythema, bullae/crepitus → necrotizing fasciitis.

5. Mucosal erosions, targetoid lesions, epidermal detachment (Nikolsky +), fever → SJS/TEN (drug reaction).

6. Diffuse erythroderma with hypotension/fever → toxic shock syndrome (TSS).

7. Urticaria/angioedema + respiratory compromise/hypotension → anaphylaxis.

8. V1 shingles (herpes zoster ophthalmicus) → risk to vision; vesicles on tip of nose (Hutchinson sign).

9. Measles-like illness (fever, cough, coryza, conjunctivitis, Koplik spots) → airborne isolate & notify

public health.

HISTORY & EXAM

1. Onset & tempo (hours vs days), migration, pain vs pruritus, fever/systemic symptoms, sick contacts/travel/ticks, new meds in last 2–8 weeks (sulfonamides, anticonvulsants, allopurinol, antibiotics, NSAIDs), vaccines, products (soaps/dyes).

2. Past hx: immunosuppression, pregnancy, cardiac/renal/hepatic disease, prior drug eruptions.

3. Exam: vitals; blanching test (glass test); mucosa (oral, ocular, genital); distribution (palms/soles involvement, dermatomal), morphology (macules/papules/vesicles/bullae/pustules/purpura), lymph nodes. Document with photos and body surface area (%BSA).

DIFFERENTIAL DIAGNOSIS (TOP 5)

1. SJS/TEN (severe mucocutaneous drug reaction).

2. Necrotizing fasciitis (rapidly progressive soft-tissue infection).

3. Meningococcemia/other invasive meningococcal disease (febrile petechiae/purpura).

4. DRESS (drug reaction with eosinophilia and systemic symptoms).

5. RMSF/other rickettsioses (fever + petechial rash, wrists/ankles → trunk/palms/soles).

INVESTIGATIONS (POC/LABS/IMAGING)

1. Unstable/'red flag' → send to ED; if delayed and scope allows, draw blood cultures and start empiric therapy (see below).

2. Stable but concerning: CBC (eosinophils, leukopenia), CMP (LFT/Cr), CRP/ESR; creatine kinase if myonecrosis suspected; urinalysis (hematuria/proteinuria in vasculitis).

3. Infectious: throat swab (scarlet fever), VZV/HSV PCR from vesicles, measles/varicella PCR per public health, RPR if secondary syphilis possible.

4. Consider skin biopsy (dermatology) for vasculitis/SJS-TEN/unclear diagnoses.

5. Avoid routine urine 'for UTI' without symptoms in older adults presenting with delirium + rash (overdiagnosis risk).

MANAGEMENT (NON-PHARM → MEDS → PROCEDURES)

A. NON-PHARMACOLOGIC

1. Stabilize ABCs; remove/stop all potential culprit drugs started in past 2–8 weeks (keep list).

2. Infection control: airborne precautions for suspected measles/varicella; contact precautions for bullous/ulcerative lesions.

3. Mark borders of spreading cellulitis; analgesia; cool compresses for pruritus; hydrate; wound care for

blisters/erosions.

4. Immediate ophthalmology if ocular involvement (SJS/ TEN, HZO). Notify public health for measles/varicella or other notifiable exanthems.

B. MEDICATIONS (EXAMPLES; INDIVIDUALIZE; CHECK ALLERGIES/RENAL DOSING)

1. Anaphylaxis: epinephrine 0.3–0.5 mg IM (1 mg/mL) anterolateral thigh; repeat q5–15 min as needed; add airway/oxygen/IV fluids; adjuncts (H1/H2 blockers, corticosteroid) after epinephrine.

2. SJS/TEN: stop all suspect meds; urgent ED/ICU/Burn referral; supportive care (fluids, wound, pain), ocular care; avoid re-challenge. (Systemic therapies vary — specialist-driven).

3. Necrotizing fasciitis: urgent ED/surgery; broad IV antibiotics (e.g., piperacillin-tazobactam + vancomycin + clindamycin) pending cultures.

4. Meningococcemia with purpura + fever: urgent ED; if delay and scope allows, give ceftriaxone 2 g IV/IM (child 50 mg/kg) then transfer.

5. RMSF suspected: doxycycline 100 mg PO/IV BID for adults and children of ALL ages (start empirically; do not wait for tests).

6. Cellulitis/erysipelas (without systemic toxicity): cephalexin 500 mg QID 5–7 d; penicillin VK for classic erysipelas; MRSA risk: doxycycline or TMP-SMX PLUS cephalexin; severe/systemic → ED.

7. Herpes zoster: start within 72 h — valacyclovir 1 g PO

TID × 7 d (or acyclovir 800 mg five-times daily); HZO or disseminated → ED/IV acyclovir.

8. DRESS: stop offending drug; hospitalize if systemic involvement; consider systemic corticosteroids (e.g., prednisone 0.5–1 mg/kg/d) with specialist guidance; monitor LFT/Cr/eosinophils.

C. PROCEDURES

1. Incision & drainage for fluctuant abscesses (send culture) unless contraindicated; avoid I&D in facial danger triangle without backup.

2. Skin biopsy if diagnosis unclear or vasculitis/SJS-TEN suspected (coordinate with dermatology).

DISPOSITION (DISCHARGE/OBSERVE/ TRANSFER) & RETURN PRECAUTIONS

1. Immediate ED/transfer: hemodynamic instability; rapidly progressive painful rash; necrosis/violaceous bullae; mucosal erosions with systemic symptoms; febrile petechiae/purpura; suspected measles/varicella in pregnancy or immunocompromised; HZO.

2. Observe/urgent consultation: uncertain diagnosis with systemic features (fever, hypotension), widespread drug eruption, immunocompromised host, infants/ elderly with dehydration risk.

3. Discharge only if stable and diagnosis benign with clear follow-up (24–72 h) and written return precautions.

4. Return immediately for: new fever, spreading redness, severe pain, dyspnea, vomiting, syncope, eye pain/ vision changes, confusion.

PEARLS & PITFALLS

1. Pain out of proportion and rapidly progressive lesions are more worrisome than 'angry-looking' but non-tender rashes.

2. Treat RMSF empirically with doxycycline — do not await confirmatory testing, including in children.

3. Non-blanching rash with fever is meningococcemia until proven otherwise.

4. SJS/TEN often starts with fever and sore throat/eyes 1–3 days before rash; check for mucosal involvement at three sites (oral, ocular, genital).

5. Avoid steroids/antibiotics 'just in case' for undifferentiated rashes; they may worsen infections or mask severity — except when indicated (e.g., anaphylaxis adjuncts, DRESS under specialist guidance).

REFERENCES

1. AAFP. The Generalized Rash: Part I & II; Evaluating the Febrile Patient with a Rash; and Dangerous Rashes in Primary Care (open articles). aafp.org

2. CDC. Meningococcal disease (clinical), Rocky Mountain Spotted Fever, Measles, Varicella, and Shingles (clinical overviews). cdc.gov

3. IDSA. 2014 Practice Guidelines for Skin and Soft Tissue Infections — open access summary. idsociety. org

4. DermNet NZ. SJS/TEN, DRESS, vasculitis, cellulitis, shingles — clinical overviews (public). dermnetnz.org

5. NICE CKS. Cellulitis and erysipelas; Shingles; Urticaria/Angioedema (public). cks.nice.org.uk

6. Emergency Care BC. SJS/TEN; Necrotizing Fasciitis — clinical summaries (public). emergencycarebc.ca

COMMON SKIN CONDITIONS — ECZEMA/PSORIASIS • SCABIES • HIVES; SKIN CANCER DETECTION

OVERVIEW & "DON'T MISS"

1. Eczema (atopic dermatitis): pruritic, eczematous patches/plaques in flexures; impaired skin barrier; flares with irritation/allergens/infection.

2. Psoriasis: well-demarcated erythematous plaques with silvery scale (extensors/scalp); consider psoriatic arthritis (joint pain/stiffness, dactylitis).

3. Scabies: intense nocturnal pruritus; burrows in web spaces, wrists, waistline, genitals; household involvement common.

4. Hives (urticaria): transient pruritic wheals (<24 h each); chronic urticaria = >6 wks; rule out angioedema/anaphylaxis.

5. Skin cancer detection: look for 'ugly duckling' or ABCDE (Asymmetry, Border, Color, Diameter ≥6 mm, Evolution) and EFG (Elevated/Firm/Growing) nodular melanomas.

6. DON'T MISS: erythroderma, eczema herpeticum, secondary bacterial infection/cellulitis, crusted scabies (hyperkeratotic, highly contagious), anaphylaxis with hives/angioedema, and suspicious pigmented/ non-healing lesions (melanoma/SCC/BCC).

HISTORY & EXAM

1. Onset, chronicity, triggers (soaps, detergents, wool, sweating, illness/meds), occupational/household exposures, travel/contact with itchy persons (scabies), systemic symptoms (fever, weight loss).

2. Distribution: flexural vs extensor vs scalp/nails; burrows/vesicles in web spaces; urticaria timing (<24 h), dermographism; photosensitivity; non-healing or bleeding lesions; 'ugly duckling'.

3. Comorbidities: asthma/allergic rhinitis; PsA symptoms (morning stiffness, swollen joints); immunosuppression; pregnancy/lactation.

4. Exam: full-skin check when feasible; lymph nodes if infection; vitals if systemic illness; measure BSA/ severity (EASI for eczema, PASI/BSA for psoriasis— optional).

DIFFERENTIAL DIAGNOSIS (TOP 5)

1. Atopic dermatitis vs contact dermatitis (allergic/irritant).

2. Psoriasis vs seborrheic dermatitis vs tinea corporis/ capitis (KOH).

3. Scabies vs bedbugs/lice vs dermatitis herpetiformis.

4. Urticaria vs urticarial vasculitis (lesions >24 h, bruise/pain) vs mast cell activation.

5. Benign nevi/seborrheic keratoses vs melanoma/BCC/SCC/AK.

INVESTIGATIONS (POC/LABS/IMAGING)

1. Mostly clinical. Consider:

2. KOH scraping (tinea) when diagnosis uncertain; bacterial culture if oozing crusts; HSV PCR if eczema herpeticum suspected.

3. Scabies confirmation: dermoscopy or mineral-oil skin scraping (mites/eggs/feces).

4. Urticaria: minimal labs; consider CBC, TSH only if chronic/refractory or guided by history; C4/tryptase if angioedema patterns suggest.

5. Suspicious lesions: dermoscopy (if trained) and prompt biopsy/referral.

MANAGEMENT (NON-PHARM → MEDS → PROCEDURES)

A. ECZEMA (ATOPIC DERMATITIS)

1. Skin care: daily lukewarm baths/showers; fragrance-free cleansers; liberal emollients (ointments/creams) twice daily and after bathing; avoid triggers; cotton clothing; short nails.

2. Topical anti-inflammatories: use by severity/site

3. Low-potency steroid (hydrocortisone 1%/2.5%) for

face/folds/infants; medium (triamcinolone 0.1%) for trunk/limbs; high (clobetasol/betamethasone dipropionate) short courses for severe lichenified plaques; step down when controlled.

4. Steroid-sparing: tacrolimus 0.03–0.1% or pimecrolimus 1% for sensitive areas/maintenance; crisaborole 2% for mild–moderate (cost).

5. Adjuncts: antihistamines for sleep itch (sedating HS as needed); treat impetiginization (topical/oral anti-staph). Bleach baths (¼–½ cup household bleach in full tub twice weekly) may reduce infections in recurrent cases.

6. Escalate/refer: phototherapy; systemic agents (dupilumab, JAK inhibitors) via dermatology.

B. PSORIASIS (LIMITED PLAQUE DISEASE IN PRIMARY CARE)

1. Education: chronic relapsing; avoid trauma (Koebner), smoking, excess alcohol; screen for PsA (joint pain/ stiffness, dactylitis).

2. Topicals: high-potency corticosteroid for plaques (e.g., clobetasol short bursts) ± calcipotriene (vitamin D analog) or fixed combos; for scalp, consider solutions/ foams/shampoos; tar/salicylic acid keratolytics as adjuncts.

3. Avoid routine oral steroids (rebound risk); consider phototherapy or systemic/biologic via dermatology for moderate–severe or special sites (face/genitals, nails, widespread).

C. SCABIES

1. Treatment of patient AND close contacts simultaneously, regardless of symptoms; environmental decontamination: wash clothing/ bedding/towels in hot water/dryer or seal in bag ≥72 h; vacuum furniture.

2. First-line topical: permethrin 5% cream neck-to-toes (include under nails, genitalia); leave 8–14 h then rinse; repeat in 7–14 days. Safe in pregnancy and infants ≥2 months.

3. Oral ivermectin (200 mcg/kg) day 1 and repeat day 8 (with food) for outbreaks, treatment failures, or crusted scabies (often multiple doses e.g., days 1,2,8,9,15 with specialist). Avoid in pregnancy/children <15 kg (consult).

4. Pruritus may persist 2–4 weeks post-treatment ('post-scabetic itch') — use emollients, mild steroids, antihistamines; ensure proper decontamination and retreat contacts if new burrows/lesions appear.

D. URTICARIA (HIVES) ± ANGIOEDEMA

1. Identify/avoid triggers (infections, NSAIDs, heat, pressure, foods/latex, stress). Assess for anaphylaxis (airway/breathing/circulation); prescribe epinephrine autoinjector if anaphylaxis history or high risk.

2. First-line: non-sedating H1 antihistamines (cetirizine/ loratadine/fexofenadine) daily; uptitrate up to 4× standard dose for chronic urticaria as needed.

3. Short course oral steroids (e.g., 0.5 mg/kg/day prednisone ≤5–7 days) only for severe acute flares not controlled by antihistamines.

4. Refractory chronic urticaria → add omalizumab or cyclosporine under specialist care. Consider H2 blocker or leukotriene receptor antagonist as adjuncts (modest benefit).

5. Pregnancy/lactation: cetirizine/loratadine preferred; avoid high-risk meds.

E. SKIN CANCER DETECTION (PRIMARY-CARE SCOPE)

1. Teach ABCDE and 'ugly duckling' self-checks; risk: sunburns/tanning beds, fair skin, many/atypical nevi, immunosuppression, FHx melanoma.

2. Urgent dermatology/biopsy: evolving pigmented lesion; new rapidly growing firm nodular lesion; non-healing ulcer/bleeding lesion; any lesion with concerning dermoscopy.

3. Preferred biopsy: excisional with narrow margins for suspected melanoma; shave is acceptable for superficial BCC/SCC in situ—follow local practice. Prompt referral if not comfortable performing biopsy.

4. Prevention: sun protection (shade, clothing, broad-spectrum SPF 30+, reapply), avoid tanning beds; counsel immunosuppressed patients on higher risk.

DISPOSITION (DISCHARGE/OBSERVE/ TRANSFER) & RETURN PRECAUTIONS

1. Immediate ED/transfer: anaphylaxis with urticaria/ angioedema (airway, hypotension), extensive secondary infection with systemic illness, erythroderma, eczema herpeticum (fever, painful monomorphic vesicles).

2. Urgent (days) dermatology: crusted scabies, treatment-refractory severe eczema/psoriasis, rapidly evolving suspicious lesion, severe generalized urticaria not controlled with high-dose antihistamines.

3. Return immediately for: new fever, spreading redness/ pus, worsening swelling of lips/tongue, shortness of breath/wheeze, or any rapidly changing skin lesion.

PEARLS & PITFALLS

1. Match steroid potency to site: lowest on face/folds/ diaper; limit super-potent duration; use fingertip-unit guidance and weekend maintenance plans for frequent eczema flares.

2. Treat ALL close contacts in scabies to prevent reinfestation; itch after therapy doesn't always mean failure.

3. Chronic urticaria is often idiopathic and benign; extensive lab work is usually unnecessary.

4. Do not use oral steroids routinely for psoriasis; coordinate systemic therapy with dermatology.

5. 'Evolution' is the most predictive ABCDE feature —

document baseline and change.

REFERENCES

1. NICE CKS. Atopic eczema; Psoriasis; Scabies; Urticaria — assessment/management (public). cks.nice.org.uk

2. American Academy of Dermatology (AAD). Atopic dermatitis; Psoriasis; Scabies; Hives; Skin cancer detection (ABCDE/ugly duckling) — public pages. aad.org

3. CDC. Scabies — clinical care and prevention; Sun safety resources (public). cdc.gov

4. DermNet NZ. Eczema, Psoriasis, Scabies, Urticaria, Skin cancer signs — detailed open-access articles. dermnetnz.org

5. AAFP. Diagnosis and Management of Scabies; Atopic Dermatitis: Rapid Evidence Review; Chronic Urticaria; Psoriasis: Topical Therapy (open). aafp.org

6. USPSTF. Skin Cancer Screening Recommendation Statement (public). uspreventiveservicestaskforce.org

SKIN INFECTIONS — FAMILY MEDICINE OFFICE (CELLULITIS, ABSCESS, IMPETIGO, ERYSIPELAS, PARONYCHIA)

OVERVIEW & "DON'T MISS"

1. Common community SSTIs: non-purulent cellulitis/ erysipelas (β-hemolytic streptococci), purulent infections/abscess (often Staphylococcus aureus incl. MRSA), impetigo (Staph/Strep), paronychia.

2. Risk factors: skin breaks (tinea pedis, eczema), edema/lymphedema, obesity, diabetes, IV drug use, bites, water exposure, recent trauma/surgery.

3. DON'T MISS: necrotizing soft-tissue infection (rapidly progressive pain out of proportion, skin dusky/necrotic, bullae, crepitus, hypotension), orbital cellulitis, septic arthritis/tenosynovitis, bacteremia/sepsis, immunocompromised host, periorbital/facial infections spreading to cavernous sinus.

HISTORY & EXAM

1. Onset/progression of erythema, pain, warmth, edema; fevers/chills; trauma/bites/water exposure; injection

drug use; comorbidities (DM, venous/lymphatic disease).

2. Localize: purulence/fluctuance (abscess), lymphangitis, portals of entry (toe webs), involvement of hands/face/genitals; prior MRSA; antibiotic exposures.

3. Exam: mark borders to monitor spread; assess for crepitus/skin anesthesia (nec fasc); check neurovascular status; look for tinea pedis/interdigital fissures; check regional nodes.

DIFFERENTIAL DIAGNOSIS (TOP 5)

1. Cellulitis/erysipelas (non-purulent).

2. Cutaneous abscess/furuncle/carbuncle (purulent).

3. Impetigo (non-bullous/bullous).

4. Deep vein thrombosis, contact dermatitis, gout/ pseudogout, insect bite reactions/lipodermatosclerosis (cellulitis mimics).

5. Septic bursitis/septic arthritis; herpetic whitlow (do NOT incise).

INVESTIGATIONS (POC/LABS/IMAGING)

1. Often clinical — no routine labs for mild cases.

2. POCUS ultrasound: differentiate abscess vs cellulitis; guide I&D; look for foreign body.

3. Cultures: swab/pus culture for purulent infections or if prior antibiotics, severe disease, or immunocompromised. Blood cultures rarely helpful in

uncomplicated cellulitis; consider if systemic toxicity or immunosuppressed.

4. Imaging (contrast CT/MRI) if necrotizing infection suspected, deep space hand infection, or orbital involvement.

5. Labs (CBC, CRP, BMP) for moderate–severe/systemic cases; LRINEC score is not reliable to rule out nec fasc.

MANAGEMENT (NON-PHARM → MEDS → PROCEDURES)

A. NON-PHARMACOLOGIC

1. Elevation of affected limb, rest, analgesia; warm compresses for small abscesses/impetigo; treat portals (tinea pedis, fissures).

2. Wound care: gentle cleansing; keep draining lesions covered; avoid sharing personal items; hand hygiene education.

3. Tetanus update if wound/trauma and status uncertain or due (see schedule).

B. ANTIBIOTICS (ADULT DOSING EXAMPLES; CHECK LOCAL RESISTANCE, ALLERGIES, RENAL DOSING)

1. Non-purulent cellulitis/erysipelas (target streptococci ± MSSA):

2. Cephalexin 500 mg QID OR amoxicillin 500 mg TID

(erysipelas: penicillin VK 500 mg QID or amoxicillin). Duration 5–7 days (extend if slow response).

3. Severe β-lactam allergy: clindamycin 300–450 mg QID. If MRSA risk low, clindamycin alone is acceptable; if uncertain strep coverage with MRSA agents, add amoxicillin.

4. Purulent cellulitis/abscess (I&D is primary therapy; add antibiotics if systemic signs, multiple lesions, large/ extremity with cellulitis, immunosuppressed, extremes of age):

5. TMP-SMX DS (160/800) 1–2 tabs BID OR doxycycline 100 mg BID — plus amoxicillin 500 mg TID if streptococcal coverage needed. Duration ~5–7 days.

6. Consider clindamycin 300–450 mg QID if local MRSA susceptibility adequate (watch C. difficile risk).

7. Impetigo (limited): topical mupirocin 2% TID or BID × 5 days after crust removal; extensive/epidemic: cephalexin 500 mg QID × 5–7 d; MRSA suspected → TMP-SMX or doxycycline (add amoxicillin if strep coverage needed).

8. Paronychia: warm soaks; if abscess → drainage; antibiotics only if cellulitis or systemic signs (same agents as above).

9. Recurrent MRSA: consider decolonization (chlorhexidine washes + intranasal mupirocin BID × 5 days) for households with recurrent infections.

C. PROCEDURES

1. Incision & Drainage (I&D) for abscess: adequate local

anesthesia; elliptical or cruciate incision over point of maximal fluctuance; break loculations with hemostat; irrigate; consider loose wick for larger cavities but avoid routine tight packing of small abscesses; bulky dressing; re-check in 24–48 h.

2. Paronychia: lift eponychial fold with #11 blade or needle; drain pus; partial nail plate removal for lateral abscess if needed; avoid I&D in herpetic whitlow (viral).

3. Orbital cellulitis suspicion or deep space hand infection → urgent imaging and specialty consult (ENT/ophthalmology/hand surgery).

DISPOSITION (DISCHARGE/OBSERVE/TRANSFER) & RETURN PRECAUTIONS

1. Immediate ED/transfer: suspected necrotizing infection, rapidly progressive erythema/pain with systemic toxicity, hemodynamic instability, orbital cellulitis (pain with EOM, proptosis, ophthalmoplegia), deep hand infection/tenosynovitis, failure of I&D with worsening sepsis.

2. Outpatient with close follow-up (24–48 h) for: facial/hand infections, significant comorbidity/immunosuppression, large abscess after I&D, or if adherence uncertain.

3. Return immediately for: spreading redness beyond marked borders after 24–48 h, persistent fever >48–72 h on therapy, severe pain out of proportion, new numbness/crepitus, vision changes, or vomiting/

weakness.

PEARLS & PITFALLS

1. Mark borders and photograph to track response; mild early progression may occur in first 24 h as antibiotics take effect — reassess clinically.

2. Treat interdigital tinea pedis to prevent recurrent lower-extremity cellulitis; consider compression for chronic edema/lymphedema.

3. Avoid doxycycline/TMP-SMX monotherapy when streptococcus is likely — add amoxicillin.

4. Do not incise herpetic whitlow; manage with antivirals and supportive care.

5. Consider water-borne pathogens (Aeromonas, Vibrio) after fresh/salt water exposure — choose appropriate antibiotics; animal/human bites require amoxicillin-clavulanate (see separate bite guide).

REFERENCES

1. IDSA. 2014 Practice Guidelines for the Diagnosis and Management of Skin and Soft Tissue Infections (open access). idsociety.org

2. NICE CKS. Cellulitis and erysipelas; Impetigo; Abscess; Paronychia (public). cks.nice.org.uk

3. AAFP. Skin and Soft Tissue Infections; Impetigo: Diagnosis and Treatment; Cutaneous Abscess Management (open articles). aafp.org

4. CDC. Community-associated MRSA — clinical

overview & prevention; Tetanus: wound management (public). cdc.gov

5. Emergency Care BC. Necrotizing Fasciitis; Cellulitis/ Abscess summaries (public). emergencycarebc.ca

6. WHO. Hand hygiene and wound care resources (public). who.int

WOMEN'S HEALTH (OB/GYN)

SECONDARY AMENORRHEA

OVERVIEW & "DON'T MISS"

1. Definition: absence of menses for ≥3 months in previously regular cycles or ≥6 months in previously irregular cycles.

2. Most common causes: pregnancy, functional hypothalamic amenorrhea (stress/weight loss/ exercise), polycystic ovary syndrome (PCOS), hyperprolactinemia, thyroid disease, primary ovarian insufficiency (POI), intrauterine adhesions (Asherman).

3. DON'T MISS: ectopic pregnancy (amenorrhea + pain/ bleeding), pituitary mass/apoplexy (headache/visual change), severe hyperandrogenism (rapid virilization— tumor), Sheehan syndrome (post-partum failure to lactate + hypotension), significant eating disorder or RED-S with bradycardia/osteoporosis risk.

HISTORY & EXAM

1. Menstrual hx: last menstrual period, prior regularity, contraception (IUD, DMPA, OCPs), post-partum/ lactation, recent procedures (D&C).

2. Symptoms: pregnancy symptoms; hot flashes/night

sweats; galactorrhea; headaches/visual change; weight change, diet, exercise; stress/illness; acne/hirsutism/voice change; pelvic pain; vaginal dryness/dyspareunia.

3. PMH/meds: antipsychotics/metoclopramide (↑prolactin), opioids, glucocorticoids; thyroid disease; diabetes; celiac; chemotherapy/radiation; family hx POI/fragile X premutation.

4. Exam: vitals (BMI, bradycardia/orthostasis), acne/hirsutism/alopecia, thyroid, galactorrhea, visual fields if concern, abdominal/pelvic exam for masses/tenderness; signs of estrogen deficiency (atrophic mucosa).

DIFFERENTIAL DIAGNOSIS (TOP 5)

1. Pregnancy (including ectopic).
2. Functional hypothalamic amenorrhea (low energy availability, stress, excessive exercise).
3. PCOS (hyperandrogenism + oligo/anovulation ± polycystic ovaries).
4. Hyperprolactinemia (prolactinoma, meds, hypothyroidism).
5. Primary ovarian insufficiency (FSH↑) vs uterine outflow obstruction/Asherman after instrumentation.

INVESTIGATIONS (POC/LABS/IMAGING)

1. FIRST: pregnancy test (urine or serum β-hCG). If positive with pain/bleeding → ED to rule out ectopic.

2. Initial labs (if not pregnant): serum TSH and prolactin.

3. Next step based on phenotype:

4. Suspected POI or long amenorrhea/estrogen deficiency → FSH, LH, and estradiol (off hormonal contraception ≥4–6 weeks).

5. Hyperandrogenism → total/free testosterone, DHEA-S; consider 17-hydroxyprogesterone (AM) for nonclassical CAH.

6. Metabolic screen in suspected PCOS: fasting glucose/ A1C, lipid profile; screen for OSA, depression.

7. Imaging:

8. Pelvic ultrasound for ovarian morphology/endometrium thickness; rule out structural lesions; identify polycystic morphology (supportive, not required).

9. Pituitary MRI if prolactin markedly elevated or neuro/visual symptoms; repeat prolactin to exclude macroprolactin or hook effect when very high.

10. Optional diagnostic trials (if uncertainty and after initial labs):

11. Progestin challenge (e.g., medroxyprogesterone 10 mg daily × 7–10 d): withdrawal bleed suggests estrogenized endometrium with anovulation/outflow patency.

12. If no withdrawal bleed, consider combined estrogen– progestin challenge vs imaging for Asherman/outflow obstruction.

13. Bone health: consider DXA if hypoestrogenism >6–12 months (FHA/POI).

MANAGEMENT (NON-PHARM → MEDS → PROCEDURES)

A. NON-PHARMACOLOGIC

1. Pregnancy desires first: algorithms differ for contraception vs fertility goals.

2. Functional hypothalamic amenorrhea: restore energy availability (increase calories, reduce excessive exercise), weight restoration, treat eating disorder/RED-S with multidisciplinary team; calcium/vitamin D; avoid using OCPs solely for bone health.

3. Lifestyle for PCOS: weight management (5–10% loss improves ovulation), exercise, nutrition; screen/tx metabolic risks (diabetes, dyslipidemia, OSA).

4. Medication review: reduce/stop prolactin-raising meds if possible (coordinate with prescriber).

B. MEDICATIONS (EXAMPLES; INDIVIDUALIZE & VERIFY CONTRAINDICATIONS)

1. PCOS (not seeking pregnancy): combined hormonal contraception for cycle control and hirsutism/acne; add cyclic progestin every 1–3 months if not using estrogen for endometrial protection; consider metformin for metabolic/ovulatory benefit.

2. Hyperprolactinemia: dopamine agonist (cabergoline preferred; bromocriptine alternative) — titrate to normalize prolactin and restore menses; treat hypothyroidism first if present.

3. POI: physiologic estrogen replacement (transdermal or oral) with cyclic progestin until average age of menopause unless contraindicated; counsel bone/ heart health; discuss fertility options (donor oocytes).

4. Hypothyroidism/hyperthyroidism: treat per guidelines — can normalize cycles.

5. Asherman/outflow obstruction: refer for hysteroscopic adhesiolysis; post-procedure estrogen + progestin to re-establish endometrium (specialist).

6. Depot medroxyprogesterone and LNG-IUD: amenorrhea is expected/benign — provide reassurance if pregnancy excluded.

C. PROCEDURES

1. Order pituitary MRI when indicated; perform/arrange pelvic ultrasound.

2. Endometrial biopsy for prolonged anovulation with risk factors (age ≥35, obesity, chronic anovulation, abnormal bleeding) or thickened endometrium.

3. Hysteroscopic evaluation for suspected Asherman (post-D&C/postpartum).

DISPOSITION (DISCHARGE/OBSERVE/ TRANSFER) & RETURN PRECAUTIONS

1. Immediate ED/transfer: positive pregnancy with pain/bleeding (ectopic concern), severe headache/ visual loss with amenorrhea (pituitary apoplexy), hemodynamic instability.

2. Urgent specialty referral (days–weeks): virilization or very high androgens (r/o ovarian/adrenal tumor), prolactin markedly elevated or neuro signs, FSH in menopausal range <40 y (POI), suspected Asherman with pain/amenorrhea post-instrumentation, refractory FHA with medical instability.

3. Return immediately for: heavy bleeding after prolonged amenorrhea, syncope, worsening headaches/vision, severe pelvic pain.

PEARLS & PITFALLS

1. Rule out pregnancy first — even if using contraception or breastfeeding.

2. Don't diagnose PCOS on ultrasound alone; use Rotterdam criteria (2 of: oligo/anovulation, hyperandrogenism, polycystic ovaries) after excluding other causes.

3. Long-term anovulation requires endometrial protection (cyclic progestin or COCs) if pregnancy not desired.

4. Macroprolactin and assay 'hook effect' can mislead — repeat prolactin with dilution if level very high and symptoms discordant.

5. Address bone health in hypoestrogenic states (FHA/POI) — weight restoration and physiologic estrogen are key.

REFERENCES

1. NICE CKS. Amenorrhoea — assessment and

management (public). cks.nice.org.uk

2. AAFP. Amenorrhea: A Systematic Approach to Diagnosis and Management (open access). aafp.org

3. Endocrine Society — Patient resources: Hyperprolactinemia; Functional Hypothalamic Amenorrhea; Primary Ovarian Insufficiency (public). endocrine.org

4. ACOG Patient Education: Amenorrhea; Polycystic Ovary Syndrome; Asherman Syndrome (public). acog.org

5. ASRM Patient Fact Sheets: Amenorrhea; Asherman Syndrome; PCOS (public). asrm.org

6. NIH MedlinePlus: Amenorrhea; Female Infertility; Polycystic Ovary Syndrome (public). medlineplus.gov

PRENATAL CARE

OVERVIEW & "DON'T MISS"

1. Goal: optimize maternal–fetal outcomes via risk assessment, evidence-based screening, immunization, and counselling.

2. Initiate prenatal care ASAP; booking visit ideally by 10–12 wks GA. Establish EDD (prefer early dating ultrasound when available).

3. DON'T MISS: ectopic pregnancy (pain + bleeding, risk factors); severe bleeding; hyperemesis with dehydration; preeclampsia (headache/vision/RUQ pain, edema, BP ≥140/90 after 20 wks); reduced fetal movement; PPROM; preterm labour; sepsis.

HISTORY & EXAM

1. Obstetric history: gravidity/parity, prior CS, preterm/ PPROM, GDM, HTN/preeclampsia, PPH, shoulder dystocia, congenital anomalies.

2. Medical: HTN, DM, thyroid, renal, autoimmune, seizures; BMI; mental health; VTE history; medications/teratogens; allergies; transfusion & blood type; Rh status if known.

3. Social: tobacco, alcohol, drugs; IPV; housing/food security; travel/exposures; occupational risks; pets (toxoplasmosis).

4. Symptoms: bleeding, pain, N/V, dysuria, pruritus/ vaginal discharge.

5. Exam: vitals incl. BP; weight/height (IOM weight-gain targets); abdominal exam; speculum if bleeding/ discharge; fetal HR after ~10–12 wks with Doppler; fundal height after 20 wks; urine dip for protein when indicated.

DIFFERENTIAL DIAGNOSIS (TOP 5)

1. Threatened miscarriage vs. ectopic pregnancy (1st trimester bleeding/pain).

2. UTI/pyelonephritis vs. asymptomatic bacteriuria.

3. Preeclampsia vs. gestational HTN vs. chronic HTN with superimposed preeclampsia.

4. Hyperemesis gravidarum vs. typical NVP; rule out thyroid & molar pregnancy if severe.

5. PROM/PPROM vs. physiologic discharge; preterm labour vs. Braxton Hicks.

INVESTIGATIONS (POC/LABS/IMAGING)

1. Initial/Booking (ideally ≤12 wks): CBC; blood type & antibody screen; rubella & varicella immunity; HBsAg; HIV; syphilis; HCV; urine culture (ASB screen); A1C or fasting glucose if diabetes risk; TSH if symptomatic/ high-risk; consider hemoglobinopathy screen by

ancestry/family history.

2. Ultrasound: dating (≈11–14 wks) if LMP uncertain or for NT if selected; anatomic scan at 18–22 wks.

3. Genetic/aneuploidy: discuss options (publicly funded varies by province): serum/NT screening or cfDNA (NIPT) based on risk/policy; informed consent required.

4. 2nd trimester: GDM screen 24–28 wks (1-step 75 g or 2-step 50 g/100 g per local policy).

5. 3rd trimester: repeat CBC & antibody screen (if Rh-neg prior to RhIG), GBS culture at 35–37 wks.

MANAGEMENT (NON-PHARM → MEDS → PROCEDURES)

A. NON-PHARMACOLOGIC

1. Prenatal vitamins: folic acid ≥0.4 mg daily (start preconception through 12 wks; higher-risk 4–5 mg/day — prior NTD, certain antiepileptics, pre-gestational diabetes, BMI ≥30; then 0.4–1 mg/day thereafter).

2. Nutrition: balanced diet; food safety (avoid unpasteurized/undercooked, listeria/toxoplasma precautions); limit caffeine (~≤200 mg/day).

3. Weight gain: use IOM ranges by pre-pregnancy BMI; encourage regular activity (150 min/week moderate if uncomplicated pregnancy).

4. Lifestyle: no tobacco, alcohol, or recreational drugs; offer cessation supports. Screen for IPV and

psychosocial needs.

5. Education: medications in pregnancy, warning signs, travel (DVT/Zika), safe work practices, dental care.

B. MEDICATIONS (EXAMPLES; INDIVIDUALIZE)

1. Low-dose ASA 81 mg nightly from 12–16 wks to delivery for preeclampsia prevention in high-risk patients (e.g., prior preeclampsia, multifetal gestation, chronic HTN, diabetes, CKD, autoimmune disease).

2. Immunizations: inactivated influenza (any trimester); Tdap once each pregnancy at 27–32 wks (earlier if risk of preterm birth); COVID-19 per NACI current guidance.

3. Nausea/vomiting: doxylamine-pyridoxine first-line; add dimenhydrinate/metoclopramide/ondansetron as needed per risk/benefit.

4. UTI/ASB: treat per culture (e.g., nitrofurantoin [avoid at term], cephalexin, amoxicillin-clavulanate—avoid fluoroquinolones, tetracyclines).

5. Chronic conditions: prefer labetalol/nifedipine/ methyldopa for HTN; insulin for diabetes if needed; avoid ACEi/ARB, statins, valproate, warfarin, isotretinoin.

C. PROCEDURES

1. Rh-negative: RhIG 300 μg at 28 wks and within 72 h postpartum if neonate Rh-positive; give after sensitizing events (bleeding, procedures, trauma).

2. Cervical sampling if due for screening; swabs for STIs

if indicated; glucose testing per local pathway; GBS swab at 35–37 wks.

DISPOSITION (DISCHARGE/OBSERVE/ TRANSFER) & RETURN PRECAUTIONS

1. Routine discharge after prenatal visits with follow-up cadence: every 4 wks to 28 wks, every 2–3 wks to 36 wks, then weekly until delivery (adjust for risk).

2. Same-day review/observe: elevated BP ≥140/90 after 20 wks, ↓ fetal movement, concerning labs, persistent vomiting/dehydration, symptomatic UTI.

3. Transfer to ED/L&D: heavy bleeding, suspected ectopic or miscarriage complications, severe abdo/ RUQ pain or headache/vision changes, seizures, PPROM, preterm labour, sepsis, severe trauma.

4. Return immediately for: vaginal bleeding, leakage of fluid, contractions <37 wks, fever, severe headache/ vision changes, marked swelling, ↓ fetal movement.

PEARLS & PITFALLS

1. Confirm EDD early and use one standard throughout pregnancy.

2. Measure BP correctly; protein assessment when hypertension suspected.

3. Discuss screening choices with clear consent; consider equity/language access.

4. Plan postpartum: contraception, breastfeeding supports, 6–12 wk follow-up; OGTT <12 wks

postpartum if GDM.

5. Document safety-netting every visit.

REFERENCES

1. NICE Guideline NG201. Antenatal care (2021). Public: nice.org.uk

2. USPSTF Recommendations (public): Asymptomatic Bacteriuria (2019), Hepatitis B (2019), HIV (2019), Syphilis (2018), Hepatitis C (2020/2023), Gestational Diabetes (2021), Preeclampsia: Aspirin (2021), Rh(D) Incompatibility (2004 reaffirmed). Public: uspreventiveservicestaskforce.org

3. Government of Canada / PHAC. Pregnancy & immunization pages (Tdap in pregnancy; influenza; COVID-19). Public: canada.ca

4. NACI (Public Health Agency of Canada). Tdap in pregnancy (optimal 27–32 weeks), Influenza in pregnancy, COVID-19 vaccine guidance. Public: canada.ca

5. CDC. Group B Streptococcus (GBS) Prevention Guidelines (2020) and pregnancy safety pages. Public: cdc.gov

6. WHO. WHO recommendations on antenatal care for a positive pregnancy experience (2016). Public: who.int

7. Perinatal Services BC. Antenatal Care Pathway & provincial forms (public). Public: perinatalservicesbc.ca

8. Health Canada. Folic Acid & Neural Tube Defect prevention; Caffeine in pregnancy; Healthy weight gain

guidelines (referencing IOM ranges). Public: canada.ca

9. BC Guidelines. Prenatal Care & related perinatal guidance (public). Public: bcguidelines.gov.bc.ca

CONTRACEPTION

OVERVIEW & "DON'T MISS"

1. Shared decision-making: match method to goals, medical eligibility, and preferences (effectiveness, bleeding profile, reversibility).

2. Long-acting reversible contraception (LARC: IUDs, implant) = highest effectiveness; offer first-line to all who desire it.

3. DON'T MISS: pregnancy/ectopic (test if symptoms or >5–7 days since last unprotected sex before quick-start); severe pelvic pain/fever (r/o PID); VTE/PE symptoms on CHC; migraine with aura (CHC contraindicated); postpartum VTE risk with CHC; chest pain/ACS and stroke symptoms.

HISTORY & EXAM

1. Reproductive goals & preferences: timing for pregnancy, desired bleeding pattern, comfort with procedures, privacy concerns.

2. Medical history & MEC review: VTE history, smoking ≥35 yrs, migraine (with aura?), HTN, IHD, stroke, liver disease, breast cancer, lupus/APS, bariatric surgery,

malabsorption, meds (enzyme inducers).

3. Gynecologic/sexual health: STI risk/screening, last intercourse & protection used, LMP/cycle pattern, dysmenorrhea/HMB, prior IUD/implant/EC experiences.

4. Exam/measurements: BP before CHC; weight/BMI for counselling (not a barrier to most methods); pelvic exam only if IUD procedure planned or symptoms indicate.

5. Breastfeeding/postpartum status, post-abortion care, and need for emergency contraception.

DIFFERENTIAL DIAGNOSIS (TOP 5)

1. Early pregnancy (intrauterine or ectopic) in patients seeking contraception after unprotected intercourse.

2. Abnormal uterine bleeding etiologies (PALM-COEIN) if bleeding pattern concerning.

3. Pelvic inflammatory disease vs. cervicitis when pelvic pain/discharge present.

4. Amenorrhea from other causes (pregnancy, lactation, hypothalamic, thyroid, hyperprolactinemia).

5. Medication-induced bleeding pattern changes (progestin-only methods, LNG-IUD, implant).

INVESTIGATIONS (POC/LABS/IMAGING)

1. Urine/serum hCG if recent unprotected intercourse, symptoms, or uncertain pregnancy status (negative test + no intercourse in last 5–7 days supports

quick-start).

2. STI screen (chlamydia/gonorrhea, HIV, syphilis, hepatitis B/C) based on risk; can screen on day of IUD insertion if no PID signs.

3. BP prior to CHC; no labs required for most methods. Consider hemoglobin if HMB; consider ferritin/TSH if indicated.

4. Pelvic exam only for IUD insertion or if symptomatic; imaging not routine.

MANAGEMENT (NON-PHARM → MEDS → PROCEDURES)

A. NON-PHARMACOLOGIC

1. Counselling & dual protection: condoms for STI prevention even with other contraceptives; discuss consent/violence screening and privacy.

2. Fertility awareness methods (cycle tracking, basal body temperature, cervical mucus) — higher typical-use failure; requires motivated, regular cycles.

3. Lactational amenorrhea method (LAM): fully/near-fully breastfeeding, amenorrheic, <6 months postpartum.

B. MEDICATIONS / DEVICES (EXAMPLES; INDIVIDUALIZE USING MEC/SPR)

1. Copper IUD (T380A): highly effective; lasts up to 10+ yrs; can be used as emergency contraception within 5 days of unprotected intercourse; expect heavier

menses/cramps initially.

2. Levonorgestrel IUDs (various doses/durations): very effective; reduce HMB/dysmenorrhea; irregular bleeding first 3–6 months, then often light/amenorrhea.

3. Etonogestrel implant: very effective LARC; irregular bleeding common; safe in most MEC categories; rapid return of fertility after removal.

4. Progestin-only pills: take daily (same time for traditional POPs; drospirenone 4 mg has longer missed-pill window). Suitable when estrogen contraindicated.

5. Combined hormonal contraception (pill/patch/ring): avoid with migraine w/ aura, VTE history, smokers ≥35, uncontrolled HTN, complicated diabetes, ischemic heart disease, stroke, severe liver disease, breast cancer, <3–6 wks postpartum depending on VTE risk.

6. Injectable (DMPA): q12–13 wks; may cause weight gain, mood change, irregular bleeding; consider bone effects in adolescents/long-term use; delayed return of fertility.

7. Emergency contraception (EC): copper IUD up to 5 days most effective; ulipristal acetate 30 mg up to 5 days (Rx); levonorgestrel 1.5 mg ASAP (label 72 h; some use up to 5 days with reduced efficacy); consider BMI effects and repeat test in 3 weeks.

8. Drug interactions: enzyme inducers (e.g., certain antiepileptics, rifampin) reduce CHC/POP/implant efficacy — use copper IUD or DMPA; counsel on backup.

C. PROCEDURES

1. Quick-start: if reasonably certain not pregnant, start most methods today; schedule follow-up pregnancy test in ~3 weeks if any doubt.

2. IUD insertion: same-day if no PID signs; consider cervical screening if due; NSAID premedication; post-insertion counselling on cramps/bleeding and when to seek care.

3. Implant insertion/removal: trained provider, local anesthetic; counsel on bleeding changes; ensure availability of removal services.

DISPOSITION (DISCHARGE/OBSERVE/ TRANSFER) & RETURN PRECAUTIONS

1. Discharge most with chosen method initiated and clear instructions; arrange follow-up in 4–12 weeks or sooner if concerns.

2. Observe/urgent review: severe pain or fever after IUD insertion (r/o perforation/PID), heavy bleeding or syncope.

3. Transfer/ED: suspected ectopic pregnancy, sepsis, chest pain/SOB (r/o PE), focal neuro deficits or severe headache (stroke) on CHC.

4. Return immediately for: pregnancy symptoms, severe pelvic/abdominal pain, fever, heavy bleeding, jaundice, chest pain, SOB, unilateral leg swelling, severe headache/vision changes.

PEARLS & PITFALLS

1. Use WHO/CDC Medical Eligibility Criteria to guide safe method selection; CHC contraindicated with migraine with aura and high VTE-risk states.

2. Offer LARC first-line to all who desire contraception — ensure same-day starts when possible to reduce gaps.

3. For denser patients or difficult anatomy during IUD insertion, use ultrasound guidance or refer rather than abandon attempt.

4. Post-EC: advise abstinence or barrier for 7 days after starting hormonal method (2 days for POPs); schedule hCG in ~3 weeks.

5. Document counselling, MEC category, and safety-netting; provide written instructions.

REFERENCES

1. World Health Organization (WHO). Medical eligibility criteria for contraceptive use; Selected practice recommendations for contraceptive use (latest editions). Public: who.int

2. U.S. Centers for Disease Control and Prevention (CDC). U.S. Medical Eligibility Criteria (US MEC) and Selected Practice Recommendations (SPR) for Contraceptive Use (2024). Public: cdc.gov

3. Faculty of Sexual & Reproductive Healthcare (FSRH, UK). Clinical Guidelines (e.g., CHC, Progestogen-only methods, Intrauterine contraception, Emergency contraception). Public: fsrh.org

4. National Institute for Health and Care Excellence (NICE). Contraceptive services for under 25s; Long-acting reversible contraception; decision aids. Public: nice.org.uk

5. Government of Canada / Public Health Agency of Canada. Sexual and reproductive health resources and STI screening guidance. Public: canada.ca

6. BC Guidelines (Public). Contraception & related primary care pathways. Public: bcguidelines.gov.bc.ca

MENOPAUSE COUNSELING & HORMONE THERAPY (HRT) BASICS

OVERVIEW & "DON'T MISS"

1. Menopause = 12 months of amenorrhea after the final menstrual period; perimenopause has cycle variability and vasomotor symptoms (VMS).

2. Common: VMS (hot flashes/night sweats), sleep disturbance, mood changes, urogenital/GSM (vaginal dryness, dyspareunia, recurrent UTIs).

3. HRT is most effective for moderate–severe VMS and GSM. Consider in healthy patients <60 years or within 10 years of menopause onset after individualized risk–benefit discussion.

4. DON'T MISS: pregnancy in perimenopause; abnormal uterine bleeding needing endometrial evaluation; VTE/PE, stroke, ACS; new breast mass; severe headache with neuro deficits.

HISTORY & EXAM

1. Symptoms: frequency/severity of VMS; sleep, mood, cognition; GSM; sexual function; quality-of-life impact.

2. Gynecologic history: LMP, bleeding pattern, contraception needs, parity, prior endometrial hyperplasia/cancer, fibroids, endometriosis.

3. Medical: cardiovascular risk factors, migraine with aura, VTE/PE history, stroke/IHD, liver disease, gallbladder disease, breast/estrogen-dependent cancers, osteoporosis/fracture history.

4. Medications/substances: tobacco, alcohol; interacting drugs.

5. Exam: BP, BMI/waist; breast exam as indicated; pelvic exam if GSM or bleeding; thyroid if symptomatic.

DIFFERENTIAL DIAGNOSIS (TOP 5)

1. Thyroid dysfunction (TSH).

2. Medication effects (e.g., SSRIs/SNRIs, tamoxifen) causing sweating/flushes.

3. Pregnancy/perimenopausal anovulatory bleeding vs. other AUB causes (PALM-COEIN).

4. Anxiety/panic, sleep apnea, infection/fever causes of night sweats.

5. Carcinoid/NET or pheochromocytoma if atypical features (rare).

INVESTIGATIONS (POC/LABS/IMAGING)

1. Diagnosis is clinical — routine FSH not required. Consider if age <45 with menopausal symptoms/ amenorrhea.

2. Before HRT: BP, BMI, CVD risk assessment; ensure

age-appropriate breast/cervical screening; pregnancy test if uncertain status; baseline lipids/A1C if risk.

3. AUB: pregnancy test; CBC; TSH if indicated; endometrial assessment (TVUS ± biopsy) per age/risk and bleeding pattern.

4. GSM: no labs needed; consider STI testing based on risk.

MANAGEMENT (NON-PHARM → MEDS → PROCEDURES)

A. NON-PHARMACOLOGIC

1. Lifestyle: layered clothing, cooling techniques, paced respiration, sleep hygiene, weight management, exercise.

2. Cognitive behavioral therapy and mindfulness can improve VMS bother/sleep.

3. For GSM: vaginal moisturizers (2–3×/wk) and lubricants for intercourse; pelvic floor therapy as needed.

B. MEDICATIONS (EXAMPLES; INDIVIDUALIZE WITH SHARED DECISION-MAKING)

1. Systemic HRT — Indications: bothersome VMS in patients <60 or within 10 yrs of menopause, without contraindications; consider bone protection benefit.

2. Contraindications: breast or estrogen-dependent cancer, active/history of VTE/PE or stroke, known IHD,

unexplained vaginal bleeding, active liver disease, known thrombophilia (unless specialist-guided).

3. Route/formulations: transdermal 17β-estradiol (e.g., 25–100 μg/day patch) has lower VTE risk vs. oral; oral estradiol 0.5–2 mg/day; conjugated estrogens per product.

4. Endometrial protection (if uterus): micronized progesterone 100 mg PO nightly (continuous) or 200 mg nightly for 12–14 days each month (cyclic); or LNG-IUS 52 mg; avoid unopposed estrogen.

5. GSM first-line: low-dose vaginal estrogen (tablet, ring, cream) — minimal systemic absorption; consider vaginal DHEA; non-hormonal options if estrogen is contraindicated.

6. Non-hormonal for VMS: SSRIs/SNRIs (e.g., paroxetine 7.5–10 mg HS, venlafaxine 37.5–75 mg/day), gabapentin 300–900 mg HS, clonidine 0.05–0.1 mg BID (less effective).

7. Counselling: use lowest effective dose; reassess 3 months, then 6–12 months; no mandatory stop age — continue if benefits outweigh risks and patient prefers.

C. PROCEDURES

1. None routine. Consider endometrial biopsy for persistent AUB; insert LNG-IUS for endometrial protection and bleeding control when appropriate.

DISPOSITION (DISCHARGE/OBSERVE/ TRANSFER) & RETURN PRECAUTIONS

1. Discharge most with counselling, shared decision, and follow-up in 3 months (earlier if side effects).

2. Urgent assessment: heavy/prolonged bleeding on HRT, new focal neurologic deficit, chest pain/ACS, SOB/leg swelling (VTE), jaundice/severe RUQ pain.

3. Adjust/stop therapy if adverse effects (migraine with aura onset on CHC-like dosing, uncontrolled HTN on oral estrogen, significant breast tenderness/bleeding).

PEARLS & PITFALLS

1. Transdermal estradiol + micronized progesterone generally has a more favorable VTE/metabolic profile than oral estrogen + synthetic progestins.

2. Do not use HRT for primary prevention of CVD, dementia, or chronic disease.

3. For high triglycerides, migraines, gallbladder disease, or high VTE risk, prefer transdermal over oral.

4. GSM often persists/worsens with age — topical therapy can be continued long-term with periodic review.

5. Always re-check need for contraception until 12 months of amenorrhea if ≥50 years (24 months if <50).

REFERENCES

1. NICE Guideline NG23. Menopause: diagnosis and management (public). nice.org.uk

2. U.S. Preventive Services Task Force (USPSTF). Hormone Therapy for the Primary Prevention of Chronic Conditions in Postmenopausal Persons (2022). uspreventiveservicestaskforce.org

3. British Menopause Society (BMS). HRT prescribing & safety updates (open guidance and tools). thebms.org. uk

4. Government of Canada / PHAC / Health Canada. Menopause & HRT safety communications and public resources (open). canada.ca

5. World Health Organization (WHO). Recommendations on menopausal care and non-hormonal options (public). who.int

MENORRHAGIA / HEAVY MENSTRUAL BLEEDING

OVERVIEW & "DON'T MISS"

1. Definition: excessive menstrual blood loss that interferes with quality of life (do not rely solely on mL). Consider PALM-COEIN classification (Structural: Polyp, Adenomyosis, Leiomyoma, Malignancy/Hyperplasia; Non-structural: Coagulopathy, Ovulatory dysfunction, Endometrial, Iatrogenic, Not otherwise classified).

2. Common causes: anovulatory cycles (adolescents/perimenopause, PCOS, thyroid), fibroids/polyps, copper IUD, anticoagulants, bleeding disorders (e.g., von Willebrand disease), adenomyosis.

3. DON'T MISS: pregnancy-related bleeding (miscarriage/ectopic), hemodynamic instability/severe anemia, endometrial hyperplasia/cancer (≥45 y or risk of unopposed estrogen), retained products post-pregnancy, pelvic infection.

HISTORY & EXAM

1. Bleeding pattern: cycle length, duration, flooding/clots, intermenstrual/postcoital bleeding, dysmenorrhea, bulk symptoms (pressure/urinary).

2. Gynecologic/obstetric: pregnancies, miscarriages, deliveries, contraception (copper IUD ↑ bleeding), prior procedures (D&C, C-section), cervical screening up to date.

3. Bleeding diathesis screen: easy bruising/epistaxis, heavy postpartum/operative bleeding, family history; anticoagulants/antiplatelets/SSRI use.

4. Medical: thyroid disease, liver/kidney disease, PCOS, obesity (unopposed estrogen), diabetes.

5. Exam: vitals/orthostatics; conjunctival pallor; BMI; pelvic exam (speculum/bimanual) for masses, cervical lesions or infection signs.

DIFFERENTIAL DIAGNOSIS (TOP 5)

1. Uterine fibroids (leiomyomas) ± submucosal; endometrial polyps.

2. Ovulatory dysfunction (adolescence, perimenopause, PCOS, thyroid).

3. Adenomyosis (globular tender uterus, dysmenorrhea).

4. Coagulopathy/anticoagulants (e.g., vWD).

5. Endometrial hyperplasia/malignancy (age ≥45, obesity, chronic anovulation).

INVESTIGATIONS (POC/LABS/IMAGING)

1. Pregnancy test for ALL reproductive-age patients.

2. CBC (± ferritin) for anemia; TSH if symptoms/risk; STI testing if cervicitis suspected.

3. Bleeding d/o screen if history suggests (adolescents, FHx, surgical/PPH bleeding): CBC, PT/INR, aPTT; consider vWF antigen/activity ± hematology referral.

4. Pelvic ultrasound (transvaginal preferred) to assess endometrium and structural causes; saline infusion sonohysterography or office hysteroscopy if intracavitary lesion suspected.

5. Endometrial biopsy: age ≥45; or <45 with risk (obesity, PCOS/chronic anovulation, tamoxifen), failed medical therapy, or persistent IMB/postcoital bleeding.

6. Cervical screening per program (not a diagnostic test for HMB but keep up-to-date).

MANAGEMENT (NON-PHARM → MEDS → PROCEDURES)

A. NON-PHARMACOLOGIC

1. Iron therapy for IDA: target ~45–65 mg elemental iron/day (or every other day) with vitamin C; IV iron for severe intolerance/malabsorption or late pregnancy.

2. Lifestyle: weight management for anovulation/PCOS; manage thyroid disease; track cycles; discuss contraception goals.

3. Avoid NSAIDs if bleeding disorder suspected until

clarified; otherwise NSAIDs help (see below).

B. MEDICATIONS (EXAMPLES; VERIFY CONTRAINDICATIONS/INTERACTIONS)

1. First-line long-term (no pathology; contraception acceptable): LNG-IUS 52 mg — most effective ($\downarrow$ blood loss ~70–90%), improves dysmenorrhea; counsel on insertion and irregular spotting initially.

2. COCs (monophasic 30–35 μg EE) cyclic or extended/continuous; reduces flow and dysmenorrhea. Contraindications per MEC.

3. Tranexamic acid 1 g PO TID (max 4 g/day) during menses up to 5 days; avoid in active/hx thromboembolism; caution with combined hormonal contraception if high VTE risk.

4. NSAIDs during menses: mefenamic acid 500 mg TID or naproxen 500 mg BID then 250 mg q6–8h; reduces prostaglandins and pain (avoid if peptic ulcer/renal risk).

5. Cyclic/continuous progestins: norethindrone acetate 5 mg TID days 5–26 or continuous; or medroxyprogesterone 10 mg daily days 5–26; DMPA may induce amenorrhea over time.

6. Fibroids/bridging to surgery: short-term GnRH agonist/antagonist to shrink fibroids and correct anemia (specialist-directed).

ACUTE HEAVY UTERINE BLEEDING (HEMODYNAMICALLY STABLE)

1. High-dose COC: one pill (30–35 μg EE) TID for 3 days → BID for 3 days → daily for 3 weeks; then standard regimen.

2. OR high-dose progestin: medroxyprogesterone 20 mg PO TID for 7 days then daily for 3 weeks; or norethindrone acetate 5 mg TID similarly.

3. Add tranexamic acid if not contraindicated; antiemetic with high-dose estrogen/progestin; recheck Hb/iron.

4. If unstable/heavy with syncope, orthostasis, or Hb very low → ED for IV fluids, possible IV estrogen, transfusion, uterine tamponade and urgent GYN.

C. PROCEDURES

1. LNG-IUS insertion (office).

2. Hysteroscopic polypectomy/myomectomy for focal lesions; endometrial ablation for completed childbearing (needs reliable contraception after).

3. Myomectomy or uterine artery embolization for fibroids (fertility counseling); hysterectomy definitive for refractory cases or malignancy/hyperplasia per GYN.

DISPOSITION (DISCHARGE/OBSERVE/ TRANSFER) & RETURN PRECAUTIONS

1. Immediate ED/transfer: hemodynamic instability, soaking ≥1 pad/tampon per hour for >2 h, syncope/ chest pain/SOB, pregnancy with heavy bleeding, fever with severe pelvic pain.

2. Urgent GYN (days): structural lesion on imaging,

failed first-line meds, anemia unresponsive to iron, endometrial biopsy indicated, suspected bleeding disorder.

3. Return immediately for: worsening bleeding, dizziness/syncope, severe pain, new foul discharge/fever after procedures or IUD insertion.

PEARLS & PITFALLS

1. Always do a pregnancy test regardless of contraception status.

2. LNG-IUS is the most effective long-term primary-care option for HMB without major pathology.

3. Endometrial biopsy threshold: ≥45 y or risk factors (obesity/PCOS/unopposed estrogen), failed therapy, or persistent intermenstrual/postcoital bleeding.

4. Copper IUD can worsen HMB — consider switch to LNG-IUS if contraception desired.

5. Treat iron deficiency even if Hb is normal (low ferritin). Recheck Hb/ferritin after 6–8 weeks.

REFERENCES

1. NICE Guideline NG88. Heavy menstrual bleeding: assessment and management (public). nice.org.uk

2. NICE CKS. Menorrhagia (Heavy menstrual bleeding) — assessment and management (public). cks.nice.org.uk

3. AAFP. Abnormal Uterine Bleeding in Premenopausal Women; Heavy Menstrual Bleeding: Evaluation and

Treatment (open articles). aafp.org

4. FIGO. PALM-COEIN classification overview (public). figo.org

5. ACOG Patient Education. Heavy Menstrual Bleeding; Endometrial Hyperplasia; Fibroids; Endometrial Ablation (public). acog.org

6. WHO. Medical eligibility criteria for contraceptive use — summaries for LNG-IUS/COCs/POPs (public). who. int

PEDIATRICS

PEDIATRIC GASTROENTERITIS (OUTPATIENT/ED TRIAGE)

OVERVIEW & "DON'T MISS"

1. Acute gastroenteritis (AGE) = acute onset vomiting ± diarrhea, usually viral (rotavirus, norovirus, adenovirus). Most are mild–moderate and managed with oral rehydration therapy (ORT).

2. DON'T MISS: moderate–severe dehydration/shock, bilious or bloody emesis, severe abdominal pain/distension, projectile non-bilious emesis (pyloric stenosis in 2–8 wks), intussusception (colicky pain, currant-jelly stool, lethargy), appendicitis, HUS with bloody diarrhea (avoid antibiotics/antimotility in suspected STEC), sepsis/meningitis in infants, DKA (polyuria/polydipsia/weight loss), UTI, surgical abdomen.

HISTORY & EXAM

1. Duration; stool frequency/volume/blood/mucus; vomiting frequency/bilious; urine output; oral intake; weight change; fever; exposures (contacts/outbreaks/

travel/food), antibiotic use, immunization (rotavirus), comorbidities.

2. Dehydration signs: appearance (alert→lethargic), cap refill, tears, mucous membranes, eyes/sunken fontanelle, skin turgor, tachycardia/tachypnea, urine output. Classify as none/mild (<3%), moderate (3–9%), severe (≥10% or shock).

3. Red flags: age <6 months or low weight, persistent vomiting, bilious emesis, severe abdominal pain, blood in stool, high fever, signs of shock, altered mental status.

DIFFERENTIAL DIAGNOSIS (TOP 5)

1. Viral gastroenteritis (noro/rota/adeno).

2. Bacterial dysentery (Shigella/Salmonella/ Campylobacter/ETEC; STEC with HUS risk).

3. Surgical: appendicitis, intussusception, malrotation/ volvulus, bowel obstruction, pyloric stenosis (infants).

4. Non-GI: UTI, otitis media, pneumonia, meningitis, DKA.

5. Food allergy, antibiotic-associated diarrhea (incl. C. difficile in older children).

INVESTIGATIONS (POC/LABS/IMAGING)

1. Usually none for mild-moderate AGE. Focus on clinical dehydration scale.

2. Stool testing (PCR/culture/ova & parasites) if: severe disease, dysentery/bloody stools, persistent

>7–14 days, travel/outbreaks, immunocompromise, suspected HUS/STEC (send Shiga toxin).

3. Labs (BMP/glucose) for moderate–severe dehydration, persistent vomiting, infants <6 months, or when IV fluids anticipated; check glucose to exclude hypoglycemia and DKA when indicated.

4. Imaging only if surgical process suspected (US for intussusception; pyloric US; appendicitis US ± MRI).

MANAGEMENT (NON-PHARM → MEDS → PROCEDURES)

A. ORAL REHYDRATION THERAPY (ORT) — CORNERSTONE

1. Use commercial reduced-osmolarity ORS (~75 mEq/L Na). Avoid plain water/soft drinks/juices for rehydration.

2. Mild dehydration: 50 mL/kg over 4 hours (plus ongoing losses).

3. Moderate: 75–100 mL/kg over 4 hours. Reassess frequently; consider NG ORS if poor intake.

4. Ongoing losses: 10 mL/kg for each loose stool; 2 mL/kg for each emesis (or small sips 5–10 mL every 1–2 minutes).

5. Breastfeeding should continue; resume age-appropriate diet early (avoid prolonged BRAT diet).

B. MEDICATIONS (EXAMPLES; VERIFY CONTRAINDICATIONS)

1. Ondansetron (outpatient single dose to facilitate ORT): 0.15 mg/kg PO (max 8 mg). Weight-based: 2 mg (8–15 kg), 4 mg (15–30 kg), 8 mg (>30 kg). Repeat only if vomit within 15 min.

2. Zinc (where deficiency risk is high, typically LMICs): 10–20 mg elemental zinc daily × 10–14 days for children <5 y.

3. Probiotics: selected strains (e.g., Lactobacillus rhamnosus GG, Saccharomyces boulardii) may shorten diarrhea modestly; evidence mixed and strain-specific.

4. Avoid: antimotility agents (e.g., loperamide) in young children or with dysentery/fever; routine antibiotics (except specific indications below).

5. Antibiotics ONLY for: suspected cholera with severe dehydration, confirmed Shigella (shortens illness), severe Campylobacter in high-risk, traveler's diarrhea with severe symptoms — choose per local guidance; AVOID antibiotics and antidiarrheals in suspected STEC (HUS risk).

C. IV/IO FLUIDS (SEVERE DEHYDRATION/SHOCK OR FAILED ORT)

1. Resuscitation: isotonic crystalloid (NS or LR) 20 mL/kg IV bolus over 10–20 min; repeat as needed to restore perfusion.

2. Then deficit replacement/maintenance: use isotonic solutions with dextrose as appropriate; correct electrolytes (monitor Na/K/Cl/HCO$_3$); treat hypoglycemia promptly.

3. Admit if persistent vomiting, severe dehydration, electrolyte derangements, social concerns, infant <6 months with moderate illness, or failed ORT.

DISPOSITION (DISCHARGE/OBSERVE/ TRANSFER) & RETURN PRECAUTIONS

1. Discharge when tolerating ORS, normalizing hydration, and caregivers confident with home plan.

2. Return immediately/ED for: signs of dehydration (no urine ≥8 h in infants or ≥12 h in older child; very dry mouth; no tears), persistent vomiting with inability to keep fluids, bilious or bloody vomit, severe abdominal pain, blood/mucus in stool, fever ≥39°C or <3 months with fever, lethargy/irritability, or concern for HUS (pallor ↓ urine after bloody diarrhea).

3. Follow-up within 24–48 h if moderate dehydration initially or if young infant/high-risk.

PEARLS & PITFALLS

1. ORT is as effective as IV rehydration for most mild–moderate cases and reduces ED/hospitalization; ondansetron increases ORT success.

2. Early refeeding improves outcomes; avoid restrictive 'BRAT' diets.

3. Check glucose in vomiting infants/ketotic children; don't miss DKA in adolescents with polyuria/polydipsia/ weight loss.

4. Consider intussusception in toddlers with episodic pain and lethargy; a normal exam between episodes does not exclude it.

5. Vaccination prevents disease: rotavirus vaccine series in infancy markedly reduces severe AGE.

REFERENCES

1. Canadian Paediatric Society (CPS). Oral rehydration therapy and early refeeding in children with gastroenteritis (open). cps.ca

2. NICE Guideline. Diarrhoea and vomiting caused by gastroenteritis in under 5s: diagnosis and management (public). nice.org.uk

3. WHO. The treatment of diarrhoea: a manual for physicians and other senior health workers; ORS/ORT guidance (open). who.int

4. CDC. Managing Acute Gastroenteritis Among Children: Oral Rehydration, Maintenance, and Nutritional Therapy; Rotavirus vaccine resources (public). cdc. gov

5. IDSA 2017 Clinical Practice Guidelines for Infectious Diarrhea (open access). idsociety.org

6. Cochrane & AAP resources on ondansetron and probiotics for pediatric gastroenteritis (public summaries). cochranelibrary.com / aap.org

WELL-BABY CARE & IMMUNIZATIONS; GROWTH/DEVELOPMENTAL SCREENING

OVERVIEW & "DON'T MISS"

1. Use Rourke Baby Record (RBR) across the first 5 years for evidence-based well-child care. Follow provincial/territorial immunization schedules (based on NACI/PHAC).

2. DON'T MISS: fever ≥38.0°C in infants <3 months; poor feeding/dehydration; failure to thrive (crossing ≥2 major percentiles or weight-for-length <3rd); developmental regression; cyanosis/apnea; bilious vomiting; jaundice persisting >2–3 weeks; abnormal red reflex; absent femoral pulses/critical congenital heart disease (CCHD); non-accidental injury concerns; postpartum depression jeopardizing infant care.

HISTORY & EXAM

1. Per visit: pregnancy/birth history (screen for risk factors), feeding (breast/formula; volumes; vitamin D), elimination, sleep (safe sleep: back to sleep, own sleep space, smoke-free), development/behaviours,

dental risk, safety (car seat/poisoning), social determinants/family supports, maternal mood (EPDS/ Whooley).

2. Growth: WHO Growth Charts (Canada). Measure weight/length and head circumference at each visit to age 2, then weight/height/BMI from age 2–5. Plot and trend; address rapid weight gain or faltering growth.

3. Developmental surveillance every visit; standardized screening at key ages (e.g., 18- and 24-month ASQ-3 or Looksee/NDDS; M-CHAT-R/F for autism at 18 and 24 months). Vision (red reflex/ocular alignment) and hearing (birth UNHS; monitor milestones).

4. Physical exam per RBR: head (plagiocephaly, fontanelles), eyes (RR/strabismus), hips (Barlow/ Ortolani early; ROM/asymmetry later), heart/lungs (murmur, pulses, SpO_2 if concerns), abdomen/ hernia, GU (testes descended, hypospadias), skin (birthmarks/bruising).

DIFFERENTIAL DIAGNOSIS (TOP 5)

1. Poor growth/failure to thrive: inadequate intake, feeding difficulties, malabsorption (celiac/CF), chronic disease, psychosocial factors.

2. Delayed development: hearing/vision impairment, global developmental delay/intellectual disability, ASD, cerebral palsy, language disorder.

3. Prolonged jaundice: breast milk jaundice, cholestasis (pale stools/dark urine), hypothyroidism, hemolysis.

4. Cyanosis/murmur/weak pulses: duct-dependent CHD, coarctation; anemia; sepsis.

5. Abnormal head shape: positional plagiocephaly vs craniosynostosis.

INVESTIGATIONS (POC/LABS/IMAGING)

1. Routine labs are not required at standard visits. Use targeted tests for red flags:

2. Prolonged jaundice (>2–3 wks): fractionated bilirubin ± thyroid and liver tests.

3. Faltering growth: CBC, ferritin, CMP, TSH, celiac screen (≥2 y or earlier if strong suspicion), stool/urine as guided; lactation/feeding assessment first.

4. Anemia screen at ~12 months if risk factors; lead/TB risk-based screening per local public health.

5. Newborn screens/hearing: confirm completion and follow up results. Hip US if breech or positive exam.

MANAGEMENT (NON-PHARM → MEDS → PROCEDURES)

A. NON-PHARMACOLOGIC & ANTICIPATORY GUIDANCE

1. Breastfeeding support; introduce iron-rich complementary foods at ~6 months (meat, iron-fortified cereals, legumes). Avoid honey <12 months; responsive feeding; open-cup practice; dental hygiene once teeth erupt; fluoride varnish per risk.

2. Safe sleep: supine, firm surface, room-share (not bed-share), avoid soft bedding/smoke; tummy time while awake. Injury prevention: rear-facing car seat, safe home (burns/poisons), water safety, fall prevention.

3. Parent well-being: screen for depression/anxiety and intimate partner violence; connect to community resources.

4. Infection prevention: routine childhood vaccines; annual influenza (≥6 months) and age-appropriate COVID-19 series/boosters per NACI; RSV prevention with seasonal nirsevimab where available (per province/territory).

B. MEDICATIONS/SUPPLEMENTS

1. Vitamin D: 400 IU/day for breastfed infants (consider 800 IU/day year-round in northern/high-risk populations). Formula-fed infants may not need extra unless high-risk; reassess diet at 12 months.

2. Iron: focus on iron-rich foods from 6 months. Consider medicinal iron in preterm/low birthweight or if iron deficiency/IDA.

3. Topicals: vitamin D and emollients for eczema prevention in high-risk? (mixed evidence) — prioritize regular emollient use for eczema treatment if present.

C. IMMUNIZATIONS (EXAMPLES; VERIFY PROVINCIAL SCHEDULE & PRODUCTS)

1. Typical infant series (province-specific products/timing

vary):

2. 2, 4, 6 months: DTaP-IPV-Hib (± HepB depending on combination used), pneumococcal conjugate (PCV15/PCV20 per local program), and rotavirus (2-dose or 3-dose brand-specific series).

3. 12 months: MMR; varicella; Men-C-C or Men-C-ACYW per jurisdiction; PCV booster if not given earlier.

4. 15 or 18 months: DTaP-IPV-Hib booster (timing varies).

5. 4–6 years: DTaP-IPV booster (pre-school/school entry).

6. Influenza annually (≥6 months); COVID-19 per NACI age-specific products/schedules.

7. RSV: NACI (2024) recommends nirsevimab for infant RSV prevention, with programs moving toward universal seasonal doses (availability varies by province/territory).

8. Use catch-up schedules when delayed; simultaneous administration of indicated vaccines is safe.

DISPOSITION (DISCHARGE/OBSERVE/ TRANSFER) & RETURN PRECAUTIONS

1. Emergency/transfer now: infant <3 months with fever ≥38.0°C; toxic appearance; respiratory distress/cyanosis; dehydration/poor feeding; seizures; bilious vomiting; suspicion of abuse.

2. Urgent referral (days): developmental regression or persistent delays on standardized screen; abnormal

growth trajectory; murmur with poor feeding/sweats/ cyanosis; persistent jaundice with cholestasis; abnormal eye findings/white pupil; undescended testes not descended by 6 months (refer by 6–9 months).

3. Return immediately for: decreased urine output, persistent vomiting, worsening jaundice, any new rash with fever, parental concern for safety/feeding or lethargy.

PEARLS & PITFALLS

1. Plot on WHO Growth Charts for Canada — not CDC for <19 years; assess trajectory, not single points.

2. Use standardized developmental tools (ASQ-3/ Looksee, M-CHAT-R/F) at 18 & 24 months and whenever concerns arise.

3. Do not give rotavirus vaccine after age limits (brand-specific maximum ages); contraindicated in SCID or history of intussusception.

4. Have anaphylaxis kit ready for all immunization visits; observe 15 minutes (30 minutes if previous reaction/ anxiety).

5. Document vaccines in the provincial registry; verify contraindications/deferrals (e.g., moderate/severe acute illness) and counsel common reactions.

REFERENCES

1. Public Health Agency of Canada (PHAC). Canadian Immunization Guide — Part 1: Recommended

Immunization Schedules; product-specific chapters (open).

2. NACI (PHAC). 2024 Statement on the Prevention of RSV Disease in Infants — nirsevimab recommendations (open PDF).

3. Canadian Paediatric Society (CPS). Rourke Baby Record — 2024 Edition (open); Caring for Kids: Vitamin D (public).

4. Health Canada. Nutrition for Healthy Term Infants (Birth to 6 mo; 6–24 mo) — vitamin D, complementary feeding (public).

5. WHO Growth Charts for Canada — Dietitians of Canada/CPS/CFPC/CPEG resources (public).

6. Provincial/Territorial routine childhood vaccine schedules (public health websites; check local program for product/age specifics).

PEDIATRIC TONSILLITIS • BRONCHIOLITIS/ASTHMA • CROUP • PNEUMONIA

OVERVIEW & "DON'T MISS"

1. Airway/breathing first: recognize work of breathing (retractions, nasal flaring, grunting), hypoxia, altered mental status, poor perfusion.

2. DON'T MISS: impending respiratory failure (fatigue, rising CO_2), epiglottitis (toxic, drooling, tripod), bacterial tracheitis (toxic, high fever, stridor not responsive to epi/steroids), peritonsillar/retropharyngeal abscess (muffled voice, trismus, neck stiffness), foreign body aspiration (sudden cough/wheeze/uni-lateral findings), severe asthma/status asthmaticus, dehydration/apnea in bronchiolitis, sepsis/empyaema in pneumonia.

HISTORY & EXAM

1. Onset/duration; fever pattern; cough (barky vs wet), stridor/wheeze, sore throat/dysphagia, drooling, voice change, apnea episodes, feeding/hydration, urinary output.

2. Risk: age <3 mo, prematurity/CHD/chronic lung/ neuromuscular disease, immunocompromise, incomplete immunizations, smoke exposure.

3. Exam: vitals incl. SpO_2; WOB score; hydration; oropharynx/tonsils (exudates/petechiae/uvula deviation), neck ROM; auscultation (wheeze/crackles/ focality); look for ear effusion and signs of AOM.

DIFFERENTIAL DIAGNOSIS (TOP 5)

1. Tonsillitis/pharyngitis: viral vs Group A Streptococcus (GAS).

2. Bronchiolitis (infants) vs early asthma/recurrent viral-induced wheeze (toddlers/school-age).

3. Croup (laryngotracheitis) vs epiglottitis vs bacterial tracheitis.

4. Community-acquired pneumonia (viral vs bacterial vs atypical).

5. Foreign body aspiration; pertussis; atypical wheeze mimics (CHF/vascular ring).

INVESTIGATIONS (POC/LABS/IMAGING)

1. Tonsillitis: RADT for GAS (backup culture if high suspicion with negative RADT). Do not test ≤3 y unless risk/outbreak.

2. Bronchiolitis: clinical diagnosis — no routine labs/ CXR; continuous pulse oximetry for moderate–severe illness; consider brief bronchodilator trial only if older infant/previous wheeze and reassess response.

3. Asthma exacerbation: pulse oximetry; consider PEF/ spirometry in older children when stable. No routine CXR unless focal findings/atypical course.

4. Croup: no routine imaging/labs; consider neck radiograph only if diagnosis unclear (avoid distress).

5. Pneumonia: CXR if diagnosis uncertain, severe disease, or failure to improve; viral testing (influenza/ COVID-19/RSV) if results change management/ isolation.

MANAGEMENT (NON-PHARM → MEDS → PROCEDURES)

A. TONSILLITIS/PHARYNGITIS (GAS WHEN CONFIRMED)

1. Supportive: analgesia/antipyretics; hydration; avoid aspirin.

2. Antibiotics ONLY with positive RADT/culture or strong clinical + epidemiology per local guidance.

3. Amoxicillin 50 mg/kg once daily (max 1 g) × 10 d OR 25 mg/kg BID × 10 d; penicillin V alternatives per tolerance.

4. Penicillin allergy (non-anaphylactic): cephalexin 20 mg/kg/dose BID × 10 d. Anaphylaxis: azithromycin 12 mg/kg daily × 5 d (watch resistance).

5. Adjunct: single-dose dexamethasone 0.6 mg/kg (max 10 mg) for severe odynophagia considered in some pathways.

6. Recurrent GAS/OSA: consider tonsillectomy per Paradise criteria (ENT).

B. BRONCHIOLITIS (INFANTS, USUALLY <2 Y)

1. Mainstay: nasal suction, hydration (oral/NG/IV), antipyretics, caregiver education. Avoid routine bronchodilators, steroids, antibiotics, or hypertonic saline in ED/outpatient.

2. Oxygen if SpO_2 persistently <90% (consider <92% threshold in very young/comorbid).

3. Consider one observed salbutamol trial in older infants with previous wheeze; continue only if clear clinical improvement.

4. Admit if: apnea, severe WOB, dehydration/poor intake, SpO_2 <90% on room air, very young age (<3 mo), or significant comorbidity.

C. PEDIATRIC ASTHMA — ACUTE EXACERBATION (OFFICE/URGENT CARE)

1. Mild–moderate: salbutamol via MDI+spacer 4–8 puffs q20 min × 3 then reassess; add ipratropium 4–8 puffs q20 min × 3 for moderate–severe.

2. Systemic steroids: dexamethasone 0.6 mg/kg PO/ IM once (max 12–16 mg) ± second dose 24–48 h OR prednisolone/prednisone 1–2 mg/kg/day (max 50 mg) × 3–5 d.

3. Target SpO_2 ≥92–94%; consider $MgSO_4$ IV and advanced therapies in ED for severe/status.

4. Discharge: start/step-up inhaled corticosteroid (ICS)

controller; provide written asthma action plan and spacer teaching; follow-up in 2–4 weeks.

D. CROUP (VIRAL LARYNGOTRACHEITIS)

1. Give dexamethasone 0.6 mg/kg PO/IM once (max 10 mg) for all severities.

2. Moderate–severe stridor at rest: nebulized epinephrine (racemic 2.25% 0.5 mL in 2–3 mL NS OR L-epinephrine 1:1000 5 mL) with observation ≥2–3 h for recurrence.

3. Avoid agitation; keep child with caregiver; heliox/ humidified air not routinely recommended; no routine antibiotics.

4. Admit if persistent stridor at rest after therapy, need for repeated nebulized epinephrine, hypoxia, severe WOB, or poor access to care.

E. COMMUNITY-ACQUIRED PNEUMONIA (CAP)

1. Preschool often viral — supportive care unless bacterial signs (focal findings, high fever, toxemia).

2. Outpatient bacterial CAP (immunized): amoxicillin 80–90 mg/kg/day divided BID × 5 days (extend if not improved).

3. School-age with atypical features (subacute dry cough, extrapulmonary): consider azithromycin 10 mg/kg day 1 then 5 mg/kg daily days 2–5.

4. Penicillin allergy (non-anaphylactic): cefuroxime/ cefpodoxime per weight; anaphylaxis: macrolide if atypical suspected (recognize pneumococcal coverage

gaps).

5. Admit if: SpO_2 <92%, dehydration, vomiting/inability to take PO, severe tachypnea, apnea, necrotizing pneumonia/effusion, social concerns or failed outpatient therapy.

DISPOSITION (DISCHARGE/OBSERVE/ TRANSFER) & RETURN PRECAUTIONS

1. Immediate ED/transfer: cyanosis/hypoxia, severe WOB/exhaustion, stridor at rest not responding to therapy, drooling/toxic appearance, suspected epiglottitis/foreign body, dehydration, altered mental status, apnea, sepsis.

2. Outpatient with close follow-up (24–48 h) for moderate cases started on therapy; sooner if high-risk.

3. Return immediately for: worsening breathing, persistent fever >72 h on antibiotics, poor intake/urine output, new lethargy, or any parental concern about work of breathing.

PEARLS & PITFALLS

1. MDI + spacer delivers SABA effectively with fewer side effects than nebulizer in most children.

2. Avoid antibiotics for bronchiolitis and viral upper airway disease; test/treat GAS only when indicated.

3. After nebulized epinephrine for croup, observe at least 2–3 h for recurrence before discharge.

4. High-dose amoxicillin remains first-line for outpatient

pediatric CAP; duration can be 5 days if clear response.

5. Check and update vaccines (DTaP-IPV-Hib, PCV, influenza, COVID-19) — prevention matters.

REFERENCES

1. Canadian Paediatric Society (CPS). Bronchiolitis: Recommendations for diagnosis, monitoring and management (open). cps.ca

2. CPS. Acute management of croup; Acute management of asthma exacerbations in children; Uncomplicated pneumonia in healthy Canadian children (open). cps. ca

3. NICE CKS. Sore throat (acute): antimicrobial prescribing; Croup; Bronchiolitis; Pneumonia in children (public). cks.nice.org.uk

4. CDC. Group A Strep — clinical guidance; Pediatric CAP & Influenza resources; COVID-19 (public). cdc. gov

5. IDSA/PIDS. Clinical practice guidelines for CAP in infants and children (open summaries). idsociety.org

6. AAFP. Diagnosis and Treatment of Streptococcal Pharyngitis; Bronchiolitis; Croup; Pediatric Pneumonia (open articles). aafp.org

FEVER IN INFANTS — OFFICE/URGENT CARE (≤3 MONTHS; 3–36 MONTHS)

OVERVIEW & "DON'T MISS"

1. Definition: rectal temp ≥38.0 °C (100.4 °F). Age-stratify: 0–21 d, 22–28 d, 29–60 d, 61–90 d, and 3–36 mo (immunization status matters).

2. Serious bacterial infection (SBI): UTI (most common), bacteremia/meningitis, pneumonia, osteo-articular infection. Viral illness remains common.

3. DON'T MISS: sepsis/meningitis, neonatal HSV (vesicles, seizures, transaminitis, ill-appearing), Kawasaki disease/MIS-C (persistent fever + mucocutaneous/GI), septic arthritis/osteomyelitis, abusive head trauma, dehydration.

HISTORY & EXAM

1. Perinatal: prematurity, GBS/chorioamnionitis, prolonged ROM, intrapartum antibiotics, HSV in mother/contacts. Feeding, urine output, behavior, sick contacts, travel, daycare, immunizations.

2. Medications/antibiotics given already; antipyretic

timing; appearance (toxicity), perfusion, work of breathing, rash (petechiae/vesicles), bulging fontanelle, meningismus (often absent in young infants).

3. UTI risk: age <12 mo (girls), uncircumcised boys <12 mo, prior UTI, fever without source.

DIFFERENTIAL DIAGNOSIS (TOP 5)

1. Viral syndrome (RSV/flu/COVID/enterovirus/ adenovirus).
2. Urinary tract infection (pyelonephritis).
3. Bacteremia/meningitis (GBS, E. coli; Listeria rare).
4. Pneumonia/bronchiolitis.
5. Neonatal HSV (disseminated/CNS/skin-eye-mouth).

INVESTIGATIONS (POC/LABS/IMAGING)

1. 0–21 days (ANY fever): full sepsis evaluation — blood culture, CBC ± CRP/PCT, catheterized urine UA & culture (or SPA), lumbar puncture (CSF cell count/ glucose/protein, culture ± PCR), ± LFTs and HSV PCR if concern; CXR if resp signs. Hospital admission.
2. 22–28 days: most still need full sepsis work-up and admission. Some pathways allow risk-stratified approach if well-appearing with normal inflammatory markers and negative UA — discuss locally.
3. 29–60 days: obtain UA & urine culture, blood culture, and inflammatory markers (ANC/CRP ± PCT). Use validated pathways (e.g., Step-by-Step/PECARN) to

decide on LP and disposition.

4. 61–90 days: UA & urine culture for all; further testing guided by appearance/inflammatory markers and source. Consider blood culture if ill-appearing or abnormal markers.

5. 3–36 months (immunized, well-appearing): focus on source. Obtain UA/urine culture in at-risk 2–24-mo children. CXR if tachypnea, O_2 desat, or focal chest signs; otherwise labs rarely needed.

6. General: respiratory viral testing when it will change management/cohorting; avoid bag urine cultures (high contamination). Prefer catheterized sample.

MANAGEMENT (NON-PHARM → MEDS → PROCEDURES)

A. NON-PHARMACOLOGIC

1. Stabilize ABCs; assess appearance quickly (well vs toxic). Ensure hydration; breast/bottle feeds on demand; avoid cold baths/tepid sponging.

2. Education: accurate rectal temperature technique; avoid aspirin; hand hygiene; safe sleep; when to seek urgent care (see below).

B. MEDICATIONS (EXAMPLES; INDIVIDUALIZE; FOLLOW LOCAL PROTOCOLS)

1. Antipyretics: acetaminophen 10–15 mg/kg PO/PR q4–6h (max 75 mg/kg/day). Ibuprofen 5–10 mg/kg PO q6–8h (max 40 mg/kg/day) — ONLY if ≥6 months old.

2. Empiric antibiotics (initiation typically in ED/inpatient after cultures):

3. 0–28 d: ampicillin + gentamicin (± cefotaxime where available for meningitis concerns). Avoid ceftriaxone in neonates due to bilirubin displacement.

4. 29–60 d (parenteral option for outpatient low-risk pending cultures): ceftriaxone 50 mg/kg IM/IV once daily with close follow-up; add ampicillin if Listeria risk per local guidance. If meningitis suspected → ED for IV ceftriaxone + vancomycin and LP.

5. UTI outpatient (≥2 months, well): cephalexin 50 mg/ kg/day divided q6–8h (or local first-line); tailor to local resistance.

6. HSV risk in neonate/young infant (ill-appearing, vesicles, seizures, CSF pleocytosis with negative Gram stain, maternal HSV): start IV acyclovir 20 mg/kg q8h and transfer.

C. PROCEDURES

1. Catheterized urine collection; avoid bag cultures. Lumbar puncture and parenteral antibiotics are typically done in ED/inpatient settings. Arrange same-day transfer when indicated.

2. Consider single-dose IM ceftriaxone for selected 29–60-day well-appearing infants being managed as outpatient per pathway with reliable follow-up.

DISPOSITION (DISCHARGE/OBSERVE/ TRANSFER) & RETURN PRECAUTIONS

1. Immediate ED/transfer: any ill-appearing infant; age ≤21–28 d with fever; poor perfusion, hypoxia, apnea, seizures, persistent vomiting, bulging fontanelle, petechiae/purpura, dehydration, or concern for HSV/ Kawasaki/MIS-C.

2. Office discharge (selected): well-appearing 29–90 d meeting low-risk criteria with negative UA and reassuring labs, reliable caregivers, and 24-h recheck plan; well-appearing immunized 3–36 mo with clear viral source and no red flags.

3. Safety-net: written return precautions — worse appearance, poor feeding (<50% normal), fewer than 3 wet diapers/day, breathing difficulty, new rash (petechiae/vesicles), persistent fever >48–72 h or any caregiver concern.

PEARLS & PITFALLS

1. Always use rectal temperatures for infants <6 months; ear/temporal readings are unreliable in this group.

2. Do not rely on 'teething' to explain fever.

3. UTI is the most common SBI in 2–24 months — obtain catheterized urine when risk is meaningful.

4. In neonates, obtain cultures BEFORE starting antibiotics when possible, but do not delay treatment in ill-appearing infants.

5. Consider HSV when there are vesicles, seizures,

elevated LFTs, or maternal history — start acyclovir early.

REFERENCES

1. NICE Guideline NG143. Fever in under 5s: assessment and initial management (public). nice.org.uk

2. Canadian Paediatric Society (CPS). Management of well-appearing febrile infants 8 to 60 days old (practice point; open). cps.ca

3. UCSF Benioff Children's Hospitals. Consensus Guidelines for Febrile Infants 0–90 Days (open). medconnection.ucsfbenioffchildrens.org

4. Royal Children's Hospital (Melbourne). Clinical Practice Guidelines: Febrile child; Urinary tract infection (open). rch.org.au

5. AAFP. Management of Fever in Infants and Young Children; Evaluation of Fever in Infants ≤90 Days (open articles). aafp.org

6. CDC/WHO. Immunization schedules and pediatric infection resources (open). cdc.gov / who.int

GERIATRICS

GERIATRICS — POLYPHARMACY & DEPRESCRIBING

OVERVIEW & "DON'T MISS"

1. Polypharmacy (commonly ≥5 meds) ↑ adverse drug events (ADEs), falls, delirium, hospitalization, and non-adherence.

2. Deprescribing = supervised dose reduction/cessation to improve outcomes when harms outweigh benefits or goals of care change.

3. DON'T MISS: delirium/acute confusion; falls/ syncope; severe hypotension/bradycardia; GI bleed (anticoagulant/antiplatelet/NSAID); hypoglycemia; hyperkalemia; QT prolongation/torsades; serotonin or anticholinergic toxidrome; opioid/benzo oversedation; lithium/digoxin toxicity.

HISTORY & EXAM

1. "Brown-bag" review: capture ALL meds (prescription/ OTC/herbal), doses, frequencies, PRNs, duplicates; assess adherence and administration barriers.

2. Goals of care: life expectancy, priorities (function,

symptom relief), number-needed-to-treat vs. time-to-benefit.

3. Symptoms possibly drug-related: dizziness, falls, confusion, constipation/urinary retention, anorexia/ weight loss, orthostasis, daytime sedation, tremor, bleeding, myopathy.

4. Functional/cognitive: ADLs/IADLs, falls in past year, gait speed, MoCA/clock draw as needed; mood/sleep, pain, bowel/bladder.

5. Vitals: BP seated/standing (orthostatics), HR; weight; hydration; review renal (eGFR) and hepatic status.

DIFFERENTIAL DIAGNOSIS (TOP 5)

1. Adverse drug reaction (ADE) including drug-drug or drug-disease interaction.

2. Delirium (infection, dehydration, pain, environment) vs. dementia progression.

3. Withdrawal phenomenon after abrupt discontinuation (benzos, opioids, clonidine, antidepressants, PPIs).

4. Undertreatment/omissions (e.g., no anticoagulation in high-risk AF; no osteoporosis therapy after fragility fracture).

5. Disease decompensation unrelated to meds (HF, infection, stroke).

INVESTIGATIONS (POC/LABS/IMAGING)

1. Medication reconciliation + interaction check (include OTC/herbals); calculate anticholinergic burden (e.g.,

ACB score).

2. Labs: BMP (Na/K/Cr/eGFR), Mg, LFTs, CBC; A1C (if on diabetes meds); INR if warfarin; TSH if thyroid Rx; B12 if cognitive concerns; urinalysis only if symptomatic.

3. ECG for QTc if on multiple QT-prolonging agents or antipsychotics; orthostatic vitals.

4. Falls assessment toolkit as indicated (vision, feet/ footwear, environment, DEXA if fracture risk).

MANAGEMENT (NON-PHARM → MEDS → PROCEDURES)

A. NON-PHARMACOLOGIC

1. Shared decision-making with patient/caregiver; document indications and stop dates for each med.

2. Prioritize: stop high-risk meds first (anticholinergics, benzodiazepines/Z-drugs, antipsychotics for BPSD, opioids/gabapentinoids combo, NSAIDs in CKD/HF, duplicate therapies).

3. Deintensify where harms > benefits: tight diabetes control (avoid glyburide; relax A1C targets 7.5–8.5% based on frailty), multi-antihypertensive regimens with orthostasis, long-term PPIs without indication, statins in limited life expectancy.

4. Simplify: once-daily dosing, blister packs, med synchronization, stop 'PRNs forever'; align with renal/ hepatic dosing.

5. Non-drug alternatives: CBT-I for insomnia, physio/
    exercise for pain, constipation regimen (fiber/PEG),
    behavioral approaches for BPSD, falls prevention.

B. MEDICATIONS (EXAMPLES OF TAPER/STOP — INDIVIDUALIZE, MONITOR)

1. Benzodiazepines/Z-drugs: reduce 10–25% dose every
    2–4 weeks; slower near end; add CBT-I/sleep hygiene.

2. PPIs (no high-risk indication): step-down to daily →
    on-demand or H2RA; trial every 4–8 weeks; reinforce
    lifestyle/alginate use; test/treat H. pylori when
    appropriate.

3. Antipsychotics for BPSD: attempt taper 25–50%
    every 1–2 weeks; stop if behaviors controlled; monitor
    relapse; use non-drug strategies.

4. Opioids (chronic non-cancer pain): decrease 5–10%
    MME q2–4 weeks; add non-opioid analgesia/physio;
    offer naloxone; avoid benzo co-prescribing.

5. Gabapentinoids: reduce 100–300 mg (gabapentin)
    or 25–75 mg (pregabalin) every 3–7 days; monitor
    sedation/edema.

6. Antihypertensives: consider stopping one agent at a
    time in orthostasis/falls; recheck BP/orthostatics 1–2
    weeks after each change.

7. Sulfonylureas/insulin in older adults with hypos: switch
    from glyburide; reduce insulin complexity; consider
    DPP-4 or SGLT2/GLP-1 only if appropriate/tolerated.

8. Anticholinergics (e.g., oxybutynin, TCAs,
    diphenhydramine): taper and replace with safer

options (mirabegron, SSRI/SNRI for neuropathic pain alternatives).

C. PROCEDURES

1. Structured deprescribing protocol: identify → assess benefit/harm → plan taper → monitor withdrawal/ relapse → document and communicate to pharmacy/ caregivers.

2. Interprofessional: refer to pharmacist for medication review; involve OT/PT, social work; falls clinic when indicated.

DISPOSITION (DISCHARGE/OBSERVE/ TRANSFER) & RETURN PRECAUTIONS

1. Follow-up: phone/visit in 1–2 weeks after each change; earlier for high-risk tapers. Provide written plan and symptom diary (sleep, pain, dizziness, bowel).

2. Observe/urgent: new delirium, repeated falls/syncope, severe withdrawal/anxiety/insomnia after taper, refractory pain, uncontrolled BP/glucose.

3. Transfer/ED: chest pain/ACS, GI bleed, severe electrolyte disturbance, serotonin syndrome, seizures, life-threatening withdrawal, lithium/digoxin toxicity.

4. Return immediately for: confusion, black stools/ hematemesis, severe dizziness/falls, palpitations/ syncope, unbearable anxiety or insomnia on taper.

PEARLS & PITFALLS

1. Start low, go slow — but GO: deprescribing is active care; change one thing at a time when possible.

2. Differentiate withdrawal vs. disease recurrence; pause/slow taper rather than reversing fully if mild symptoms.

3. Use tools: AGS Beers Criteria (public summaries), STOPP/START/STOPPFrail (use accessible summaries), Deprescribing.org algorithms, ACB score, Choosing Wisely lists.

4. Mind renal dosing (eGFR) and drug-drug interactions (CYP/P-gp); review OTCs (diphenhydramine, NSAIDs).

5. Always align with patient goals; document consent, monitoring plan, and who to call for help.

REFERENCES

1. Deprescribing.org / Bruyère Research Institute — Evidence-based deprescribing algorithms (PPIs, benzos, antipsychotics, gabapentinoids, etc.). Public: deprescribing.org

2. Choosing Wisely Canada — Geriatrics & medication recommendations (public lists). choosingwiselycanada. org

3. NICE NG56. Multimorbidity: clinical assessment and management; NG5 Medicines optimisation: safe and effective use of medicines (public). nice.org.uk

4. NHS Scotland. Polypharmacy Guidance, Realistic Prescribing (7th ed. and updates) — open PDF.

polypharmacy.scot.nhs.uk

5. US Deprescribing Research Network — clinician tools & patient handouts (open). usdeprescribing.org

6. American Geriatrics Society (AGS) Beers Criteria — public summary/resources. geriatricscareonline.org (public summaries)

7. Anticholinergic Cognitive Burden (ACB) Scale — public calculators and lists. acbcalc.com / related public resources

GERIATRICS — FALLS ASSESSMENT

OVERVIEW & "DON'T MISS"

1. Falls are common and multifactorial; risk ↑ with age, frailty, polypharmacy, sensory loss, and environmental hazards.

2. A fall in an older adult warrants assessment even without injury. Recurrent falls (≥2 in 12 months) or any fall with injury → comprehensive evaluation.

3. DON'T MISS: syncope/cardiac cause (arrhythmia, aortic stenosis), stroke/TIA, subdural hematoma, cervical/hip fracture, orthostatic hypotension with dehydration/sepsis, hypoglycemia, medication toxicity (sedatives, antihypertensives, anticholinergics).

HISTORY & EXAM

1. History of the fall(s): circumstances, prodrome (lightheadedness, palpitations), activity, footwear, surface, time of day; injuries; ability to rise; fear of falling.

2. Medical history: prior falls, gait/balance problems, neuropathy, vision/hearing, continence, cognition/ depression, pain, alcohol use, sleep, osteoporosis/

fractures.

3. Medication review (prescription/OTC/herbal): psychotropics (benzos/Z-drugs, antipsychotics), TCAs/anticholinergics, opioids/gabapentinoids, antihypertensives, hypoglycemics, diuretics, polypharmacy ≥5.

4. Functional/social: ADLs/IADLs, assistive devices, home environment (rugs, stairs, lighting), supports/caregivers.

5. Exam: vitals including orthostatics (drop ≥20 SBP or ≥10 DBP within 3 min), cardiac exam (murmurs/irregular), neuro (strength, sensation, vibration/proprioception), feet/footwear, vision (acuity), cognition (MoCA/clock draw), depression screen (PHQ-2).

6. Mobility tests: Timed Up & Go (TUG) — ≥12 s suggests ↑ risk; 5-Times Sit-to-Stand (5xSTS) — ≥15 s predicts weakness/fall risk; gait speed — <0.8 m/s frailty risk; consider Berg Balance (if trained).

DIFFERENTIAL DIAGNOSIS (TOP 5)

1. Mechanical fall (environmental + deconditioning).

2. Orthostatic hypotension/volume depletion or medication-related hypotension.

3. Gait disorder: neuropathy, Parkinson disease, cerebellar disease.

4. Cardiac syncope/arrhythmia; carotid sinus hypersensitivity (rare).

5. Vestibular disorder (BPPV), visual impairment, foot

problems.

INVESTIGATIONS (POC/LABS/IMAGING)

1. Targeted: orthostatic vitals; ECG for arrhythmia/QT; capillary glucose (hypoglycemia).

2. Labs if indicated: CBC (anemia), electrolytes/renal (dehydration, hyponatremia), TSH/B12 if neuropathy/ cognitive concerns; vitamin D only if deficiency risk — not for routine falls prevention.

3. Imaging: X-ray suspected fractures (hip, wrist, vertebrae); head CT if head strike/anticoagulants or new neuro deficits; carotid imaging usually not indicated for falls alone.

4. Consider medication level/toxicity (e.g., digoxin, lithium) if symptomatic or interacting drugs.

MANAGEMENT (NON-PHARM → MEDS → PROCEDURES)

A. NON-PHARMACOLOGIC

1. Exercise/physiotherapy: multicomponent strength + balance training (e.g., Otago, tai chi) 2–3×/week; gait aid assessment and training.

2. Home/environment: remove loose rugs/clutter, install grab bars/rails, improve lighting/night lights, non-slip footwear; OT home safety assessment if available.

3. Vision/hearing: optimize acuity (glasses/cataract referral), hearing aids; avoid new multifocal lenses for

outdoor ambulation.

4. Continence: address urgency/nocturia; consider scheduled voiding; review diuretic timing.

5. Bone health: assess fracture risk (e.g., FRAX), treat osteoporosis (bisphosphonates first-line) and consider hip protectors in LTC/high-risk.

6. Education: teach 'how to rise from floor'; provide falls plan and emergency response (personal alarm).

B. MEDICATIONS (EXAMPLES; INDIVIDUALIZE)

1. Deprescribing: taper/stop high-risk agents (benzos/Z-drugs, anticholinergics, antipsychotics, opioids/gabapentinoids when possible); simplify antihypertensives if orthostasis; avoid tight glycemic control.

2. Orthostatic hypotension: non-drug first (hydration, slow position changes, compression stockings/abdominal binder, elevate head of bed, small frequent meals). If persistent & symptomatic: consider midodrine 2.5–10 mg TID or fludrocortisone 0.1–0.2 mg/day (monitor BP, supine HTN, K^+).

3. Vitamin D: do NOT start solely to prevent falls (no benefit in average-risk); replete only if deficient per local guidance.

4. Osteoporosis: calcium (dietary preferred) + vitamin D as per bone health guidelines; pharmacotherapy for high-risk/fragility fractures.

C. PROCEDURES

1. Assistive devices: prescribe cane/walker fit; PT training to use correctly.

2. Foot care: podiatry for nail/ulcer care; orthotics if indicated.

3. Referrals: PT/OT, community falls programs, optometry/ophthalmology (cataract), audiology, pharmacist medication review, geriatrics for complex/ recurrent falls.

DISPOSITION (DISCHARGE/OBSERVE/ TRANSFER) & RETURN PRECAUTIONS

1. Discharge: provide written plan (exercise, home safety, med changes), arrange follow-up in 4–12 weeks to reassess TUG/5xSTS and orthostatics.

2. Observe/urgent: recurrent unexplained falls, hypotension/syncope, new neuro findings, or suspected fracture without clear imaging access.

3. Transfer/ED: head injury on anticoagulants/ antiplatelets, suspected hip fracture (unable to weight-bear), syncope with concerning ECG, acute stroke/TIA, severe dehydration/electrolyte derangement.

4. Return immediately for: new weakness/numbness, chest pain, palpitations, severe headache, vision loss, or inability to mobilize after a fall.

PEARLS & PITFALLS

1. Ask about falls every visit in older adults; one fall

predicts more.

2. A single simple test (TUG) plus orthostatic vitals captures many high-risk patients — re-test after interventions.

3. Treat hypotension and deconditioning first; deprescribing psychotropics often yields large gains.

4. Multicomponent programs (exercise + home safety + vision + med review) work better than single interventions.

5. Document fall circumstances and a concrete plan with who is implementing what (patient, caregiver, PT/OT).

REFERENCES

1. CDC STEADI (Stopping Elderly Accidents, Deaths & Injuries) — clinician toolkit and algorithms (public). cdc.gov/steadi

2. USPSTF. Interventions to Prevent Falls in Community-Dwelling Older Adults (most recent recommendation statement; public). uspreventiveservicestaskforce.org

3. NICE. Falls in older people: assessing risk and prevention — guideline & quality standard (public). nice.org.uk

4. British Geriatrics Society. Best practice guideline for the assessment and prevention of falls in older people (open resources). bgs.org.uk

5. WHO. Step safely: strategies for preventing and managing falls across the life-course (public). who.int

6. Choosing Wisely Canada. Geriatrics & falls-related

recommendations (public). choosingwiselycanada.org

7. BC Guidelines / Provincial resources on falls risk in community-dwelling older adults (public). bcguidelines. gov.bc.ca

DELIRIUM VS DEMENTIA, DEPRESSION IN ELDERS

OVERVIEW & "DON'T MISS"

1. Delirium = acute/subacute change in attention & cognition with fluctuation and altered level of arousal; usually due to an underlying medical/medication cause — medical emergency.

2. Dementia (major neurocognitive disorder) = chronic progressive decline in ≥1 cognitive domain impairing function; attention/alertness generally preserved until late stages.

3. Depression can mimic or coexist ("pseudodementia"): reduced effort, 'I don't know' answers, worst in mornings, prominent affective symptoms.

4. DON'T MISS: stroke/TIA, sepsis, hypoglycemia, hypoxia/CO_2 retention, MI, GI bleed, intoxication/withdrawal, subdural hematoma, normal pressure hydrocephalus, suicidal ideation.

HISTORY & EXAM

1. Collateral history (caregiver): timeline (hours–days

vs months–years), fluctuation, sleep/wake reversal, hallucinations, recent illness/surgery, falls/head injury, urinary/constipation issues, pain, sensory losses (hearing/vision), medications (anticholinergics, sedatives, opioids, steroids), alcohol/benzos.

2. Screen tools (quick): 4AT for delirium (alertness, AMT4, attention, acute change); Mini-Cog (3-word recall + clock) or MoCA for cognition; GDS-15 or PHQ-2/9 for depression.

3. Exam: vitals incl. orthostatics, oxygenation; hydration; neuro (focal deficits, parkinsonism suggesting LBD), gait; pupils; signs of infection; CVD (murmur/AF). Check hearing aids/glasses fit.

DIFFERENTIAL DIAGNOSIS (TOP 5)

1. Delirium (hyperactive, hypoactive, or mixed) due to infection, medications, metabolic derangements, pain, urinary retention/constipation, dehydration.

2. Dementia types: Alzheimer, vascular, Lewy body (fluctuations, visual hallucinations, parkinsonism), frontotemporal (behavior/language), mixed.

3. Depression ± anxiety; bereavement; adjustment disorder.

4. Medication effects/toxicity (anticholinergics, benzodiazepines, opioids, polypharmacy).

5. Hypothyroidism, B12 deficiency, neurosyphilis (rare), sleep apnea.

INVESTIGATIONS (POC/LABS/IMAGING)

1. Bedside: glucose, SpO_2; ECG if arrhythmia/ischemia suspected.

2. Labs (tailor): CBC, CMP (Na/K/Ca/Cr), glucose/A1C, LFTs, TSH, B12; urinalysis only if urinary symptoms/systemic signs (avoid overdiagnosing ASB).

3. Infectious work-up as indicated: CXR if respiratory symptoms; cultures if febrile/toxic.

4. CT head: new focal deficits, anticoagulation with head strike, severe headache, persistent confusion unexplained, or stepwise deficits (consider subdural).

5. Cognitive testing baseline (Mini-Cog/MoCA) once delirium ruled out/improved; depression screening (GDS-15/PHQ-9).

MANAGEMENT (NON-PHARM → MEDS → PROCEDURES)

A. NON-PHARMACOLOGIC

1. Delirium: treat triggers ('PINCH ME' — Pain, Infection, Nutrition, Constipation, Hydration, Medications, Environment). Re-orient frequently; ensure hearing aids/glasses; mobilize early; sleep hygiene (lights off at night, avoid frequent vitals); bowel/bladder regimen; avoid restraints.

2. Dementia: care partner education; routine/structure; exercise; cognitive stimulation; address safety (driving, stove); advance care planning; treat hearing/vision

loss; manage vascular risks.

3. Depression: supportive counselling; behavioral activation; grief support; address loneliness; consider psychotherapy referral (CBT, PST).

B. MEDICATIONS (EXAMPLES; INDIVIDUALIZE & REVIEW INTERACTIONS/RENAL DOSING)

1. Delirium: avoid antipsychotics unless severe distress or risk to self/others after non-drug measures; then lowest dose/short course (e.g., haloperidol 0.5–1 mg PO/IM q4–6h PRN; avoid in Parkinson/LBD — use quetiapine 12.5–25 mg). Avoid benzodiazepines except for alcohol/benzo withdrawal.

2. Pain: acetaminophen scheduled; avoid anticholinergic agents; cautious low-dose opioids if necessary with bowel regimen.

3. Sleep: avoid z-drugs; consider melatonin 2–5 mg HS; sleep hygiene first.

4. Dementia pharmacotherapy: cholinesterase inhibitors (donepezil, rivastigmine, galantamine) may help cognition/function in Alzheimer/LBD; memantine for moderate–severe Alzheimer. Monitor bradycardia, syncope, weight loss; re-assess benefit regularly and deprescribe if no clear benefit.

5. Behavioral & psychological symptoms of dementia (BPSD): non-drug first; if dangerous psychosis/aggression, consider risperidone low dose, shortest duration; discuss stroke/mortality risks; obtain consent and plan taper.

6. Depression: SSRIs first-line (sertraline, citalopram ≤20 mg if >60 due to QT; avoid paroxetine/TCAs for anticholinergic burden). Start low/go slow, monitor hyponatremia/falls. Consider mirtazapine for weight loss/insomnia. Combine with psychotherapy. Monitor for suicidal ideation.

C. PROCEDURES

1. Hearing/vision referrals; gait/physio; home safety/OT assessment; caregiver support programs; community resources (adult day programs, Alzheimer Society).

DISPOSITION (DISCHARGE/OBSERVE/ TRANSFER) & RETURN PRECAUTIONS

1. Discharge: identifiable cause treated/plan in place, safety assured, caregiver understands red flags; arrange follow-up within 1–2 weeks (earlier if medication started).

2. Observe/urgent referral: persistent/worsening delirium, inability to ensure safety, severe dehydration/ malnutrition, suspicion of Lewy body dementia with antipsychotic sensitivity.

3. ED/Transfer: suspected stroke/TIA, sepsis, acute coronary syndrome, GI bleed, subdural, severe agitation with risk of harm, active suicidal ideation.

4. Return immediately for: new fever, chest pain, dyspnea, unilateral weakness, new falls, uncontrolled agitation, refusal to eat/drink >24 h.

PEARLS & PITFALLS

1. Delirium hallmark = inattention with acute onset and fluctuating course; hypoactive subtype is common and easily missed.

2. Treat sensory deprivation: hearing amplifiers and glasses can rapidly improve confusion.

3. Avoid routine antipsychotics for delirium — correct causes first; document indication, duration, and taper plan if used.

4. Depression can present as cognitive complaints; screen with GDS-15/PHQ-9 and treat — improvement may clarify baseline cognition.

5. Always review medications (anticholinergics, benzodiazepines, opioids, antispasmodics, antihistamines, steroids) and deprescribe where possible.

REFERENCES

1. NICE Guideline NG103. Delirium: prevention, diagnosis and management (public). nice.org.uk

2. NICE Guideline NG97. Dementia: assessment, management and support for people living with dementia and their carers (public). nice.org.uk

3. British Geriatrics Society. Delirium Guidelines & Toolkit (open resources). bgs.org.uk

4. 4AT (Rapid Clinical Test for Delirium). Official website (public). the4AT.com

5. CAM (Confusion Assessment Method) — training &

materials (public). Hospital Elder Life Program (help. agscocare.org)

6. USPSTF. Screening for Depression in Adults, including Older Adults (recommendation statement). uspreventiveservicestaskforce.org

7. NIA/NIH & Alzheimer Society (public pages) — dementia information and caregiver resources. nia.nih. gov / alzheimer.ca

8. Choosing Wisely Canada. Delirium/dementia & antipsychotic use recommendations (public). choosingwiselycanada.org

FRAILTY ASSESSMENT — FAMILY MEDICINE OFFICE

OVERVIEW & "DON'T MISS"

1. Frailty = decreased physiologic reserve and resistance to stressors, leading to vulnerability to adverse outcomes (falls, delirium, hospitalization, mortality). It is not the same as age or disability.

2. Common models: phenotype (weight loss, exhaustion, weakness, slow gait, low activity) and deficit accumulation (Clinical Frailty Scale—CFS).

3. DON'T MISS: delirium, acute infection/sepsis, dehydration/AKI, hypoglycemia, stroke/TIA, ACS/PE, hip/spine fracture, medication toxicity (anticholinergics/benzos/opioids), elder abuse/neglect.

HISTORY & EXAM

1. Functional: ADLs/IADLs, falls/past year, near-falls, mobility aids, stairs, incontinence; cognitive (memory, attention), mood (PHQ-2/9, GDS-15), sleep, pain, fatigue.

2. Nutrition: weight loss ≥5% in 6–12 months, appetite,

chewing/swallowing, dentition, alcohol; screen with SNAQ or MUST if available.

3. Social: living situation, caregivers, loneliness, finances, transportation, advanced directives/goals of care.

4. Medications: polypharmacy (≥5–10 meds), high-risk drugs (anticholinergics, benzodiazepines, Z-drugs, antipsychotics, opioids, antihypertensives causing orthostasis), duplication, adherence.

5. Exam: vitals incl. orthostatics; vision/hearing; gait/ balance; muscle bulk; edema; oral health; cognition screen (Mini-Cog) and delirium screen (4AT) when acute.

DIFFERENTIAL DIAGNOSIS (TOP 5)

1. Sarcopenia (loss of muscle mass/strength/ performance) ± malnutrition.

2. Depression, social isolation, caregiver burnout.

3. Undiagnosed cognitive impairment/dementia or delirium.

4. Multimorbidity with deconditioning (HF, COPD, CKD).

5. Reversible contributors: hypothyroidism, B12 deficiency, anemia, poorly controlled diabetes, OSA, medications.

INVESTIGATIONS (POC/LABS/IMAGING)

1. Basic labs when clinically indicated: CBC (anemia), CMP (eGFR/electrolytes), TSH, vitamin B12 (± MMA), 25-OH vitamin D, A1C, CRP if inflammatory disease

suspected; urinalysis only if urinary symptoms.

2. Screening tools (choose one primary + adjuncts):

3. Clinical Frailty Scale (CFS 1–9): judgement-based global frailty ($\geq$5 = frail).

4. FRAIL questionnaire (Fatigue, Resistance, Ambulation, Illnesses, Loss of weight) — $\geq$3 = frail; 1–2 = pre-frail.

5. PRISMA-7 ($\geq$3 suggests frailty).

6. Edmonton Frail Scale (EFS) — multidomain including cognition/timed 'get up and go'.

7. Physical performance:

8. Gait speed (usual pace over 4 m): <0.8 m/s suggests frailty/high risk; $\leq$0.6 m/s very high risk.

9. Timed Up & Go (TUG): >12 s indicates higher falls risk; $\geq$20 s significant impairment.

10. Grip strength (hand dynamometer): below age/sex norms indicates weakness/sarcopenia.

MANAGEMENT (NON-PHARM $\rightarrow$ MEDS $\rightarrow$ PROCEDURES)

A. NON-PHARMACOLOGIC (CORNERSTONES)

1. Comprehensive Geriatric Assessment (CGA) approach: address medical, functional, cognitive, psychological, and social domains; involve interdisciplinary team (physio/OT/pharmacy/dietitian/ social work).

2. Exercise: progressive resistance + balance + aerobic training 2–3×/wk; start low and progress; include

sit-to-stands, step training, and walking plans.

3. Nutrition: protein 1.0–1.2 g/kg/day (up to ~1.5 g/kg/day if malnourished/ill unless contraindicated), energy repletion, vitamin D repletion if deficient; consider oral nutritional supplements if intake poor.

4. Falls prevention: home hazard assessment, footwear, vision/hearing aids, vitamin D if low, treat orthostatic hypotension (fluids, meds review, compression stockings, slow position changes).

5. Sleep & continence: sleep hygiene, treat pain/OSA; bladder training; constipation regimen.

6. Social supports: caregiver respite, day programs, community exercise classes, transport services; discuss goals of care/advance directives.

B. MEDICATIONS (OPTIMIZE & DEPRESCRIBE)

1. Review and deprescribe high-risk meds (anticholinergics, benzodiazepines/Z-drugs, antipsychotics without clear indication, sedating antihistamines, high-dose opioids).

2. Simplify regimens (once-daily dosing, blister packs) and align with priorities (symptom relief vs disease modification).

3. Use STOPP/START or equivalent criteria to identify potentially inappropriate medications and omissions; check anticholinergic burden scales.

4. Avoid tight glycemic/BP targets if high hypo/falls risk; individualize (often A1C 7.5–8.5%, SBP 130–150 depending on context).

C. PROCEDURES/CLINIC TESTS

1. Measure gait speed (4-m walk), TUG, and grip strength; document CFS score at each visit (especially after illness).

2. Orthostatic vitals; vision/hearing screening; foot risk exam; review mobility aids fit and teach safe transfer techniques.

3. Create a written care plan with goals, exercise prescription, nutrition targets, and follow-up intervals.

DISPOSITION (DISCHARGE/OBSERVE/ TRANSFER) & RETURN PRECAUTIONS

1. ED/Immediate: suspected delirium with sepsis/acute focal deficits, syncope with injury, suspected hip/spine fracture, dehydration with hypotension, acute GI bleed, suicidal ideation, elder abuse.

2. Urgent (days): rapid functional decline (new need for help with basic ADLs), >5% weight loss in 1–3 months, recurrent falls, new incontinence with gait/cognitive decline, caregiver breakdown; consider home care/ geriatric referral.

3. Routine follow-up: re-assess function, falls risk, nutrition, cognition, mood, and meds every 3–6 months; adjust plan after any hospitalization/illness ('post-hospital frailty check').

4. Return immediately for: new confusion, inability to stand/walk, chest pain, new focal weakness/speech change, severe dehydration, or unsafe home situation.

PEARLS & PITFALLS

1. Frailty is dynamic — reassess after acute illnesses and after interventions (exercise/nutrition).
2. A slow gait speed is as predictive as many lab tests — measure it routinely.
3. Do not over-medicalize: align with patient goals; prioritize function, symptom control, and safety.
4. Screen for and treat sarcopenia and malnutrition early; small gains in strength translate to big functional wins.
5. Every medication is a 'trial' in frail adults — start low, go slow, set a stop date if no benefit.

REFERENCES

1. NHS / Dalhousie University. Clinical Frailty Scale (CFS) user guide and scale (public). nhs.uk & cfn-nce. ca (Canadian Frailty Network)
2. British Geriatrics Society (BGS). Fit for Frailty parts 1 & 2 — recognition and management of frailty in community/primary care (open PDFs). bgs.org.uk
3. WHO. ICOPE (Integrated Care for Older People) guidelines and handbook (open). who.int
4. NICE Guideline NG56. Multimorbidity: clinical assessment and management (public). nice.org.uk
5. AAFP. Frailty: Evaluation and Management; Gait Speed and Other Functional Measures; Timed Up and Go Test (open articles). aafp.org
6. Edmonton Frail Scale resources (University of Alberta) — toolkit and scoring (public). ualberta.ca (geriatrics)

7. PRISMA-7 and FRAIL questionnaire summaries —
    public tools via BGS/CFN/academic sources (public)

PSYCHIATRY & ADDICTION

QUICK OVERVIEW — DEPRESSION, BIPOLAR DISORDER, ADHD, ANXIETY, PSYCHOTIC DISORDERS & SUBSTANCE USE

OVERVIEW & "DON'T MISS"

1. Screen systematically and triage risk at every visit with mental-status + safety check.

2. DON'T MISS: suicidal/homicidal ideation or intent, psychosis with risk to self/others, severe agitation or catatonia, acute intoxication/withdrawal (alcohol, benzodiazepines, opioids, stimulants), serotonin syndrome, neuroleptic malignant syndrome (NMS), postpartum psychosis, mania with impaired judgment, delirium due to medical/toxic causes.

HISTORY & EXAM

1. Depression: mood, anhedonia, sleep/appetite, energy, concentration, psychomotor, guilt/hopelessness; screen with PHQ-9.

2. Bipolar: prior mania/hypomania (↓sleep + ↑energy,

grandiosity, pressured speech, risky behavior); family history; antidepressant-induced switches.

3. ADHD: childhood onset (before 12), functional impairment across settings; inattentive/ hyperactive-impulsive symptoms; screen (ASRS).

4. Anxiety: excessive worry (GAD), panic attacks, avoidance, OCD symptoms, trauma exposure (PTSD).

5. Psychosis: hallucinations, delusions, disorganization; assess insight, negative symptoms, cognitive changes.

6. Substance use: type/amount/pattern; screens (AUDIT-C, ASSIST/DAST-10, CRAFFT for youth); overdose/withdrawal history; readiness to change.

7. Medical review: meds (steroids, isotretinoin, interferons, bupropion/stimulants), thyroid, sleep apnea, pain, neurologic disease; vitals incl. weight/BP; mental-status exam.

DIFFERENTIAL DIAGNOSIS (TOP 5)

1. Primary mood/anxiety/psychotic disorders.

2. Substance-/medication-induced disorders (intoxication/ withdrawal; antidepressant activation; anticholinergics; steroids).

3. Medical causes: hypothyroid/hyperthyroid, anemia, B12 deficiency, sleep apnea, infections (HIV/syphilis), neuro (epilepsy, dementia, tumor), delirium.

4. Personality disorders and trauma-related conditions.

5. Normal stress reactions/bereavement — still assess safety/impairment.

INVESTIGATIONS (POC/LABS/IMAGING)

1. Screening scales: PHQ-9 (depression), GAD-7 (anxiety), ASRS (adult ADHD), MDQ (bipolar screen), PCL-5 (PTSD), AUDIT-C (alcohol).

2. Baseline labs when indicated: TSH, CBC, CMP (Na, renal/liver), B12 (± folate), A1C/lipids (antipsychotics), pregnancy test (teratogenic meds), urine tox if unclear picture; HIV/syphilis if risk.

3. ECG (QTc) if starting QT-prolonging agents (antipsychotics, TCAs, methadone) or cardiac risk; consider prolactin if antipsychotic-induced symptoms.

4. Neuroimaging only if focal deficits, head trauma, late-onset psychosis, or atypical features.

MANAGEMENT (NON-PHARM → MEDS → PROCEDURES)

A. NON-PHARMACOLOGIC (ALL CONDITIONS)

1. Safety first: brief suicide risk assessment (ideation, plan, intent, means, protective factors); safety plan; restrict means; crisis numbers; involve supports (with consent).

2. Psychoeducation and shared decision-making; sleep hygiene; exercise; regular schedule; reduce alcohol/cannabis; trauma-informed care.

3. Psychotherapies: CBT (depression/anxiety), IPT/behavioral activation (depression), exposure-based (anxiety/PTSD), family-focused (bipolar), skills

(DBT elements), organizational coaching (ADHD), contingency management (stimulants). SBIRT for substance use.

B. MEDICATIONS (PRIMARY-CARE SCOPE — INDIVIDUALIZE & CHECK INTERACTIONS/ CONTRAINDICATIONS)

1. Depression (unipolar): SSRIs (sertraline/escitalopram/ citalopram/fluoxetine) or SNRIs (venlafaxine/ duloxetine). Start low, ↑ every 2–4 wks; reassess at 4–6 wks. Augment with bupropion or mirtazapine if partial response. Continue ≥6–12 mo after remission (longer if recurrent).

2. Bipolar: AVOID antidepressant monotherapy. Acute mania/hypomania → mood stabilizer (lithium, valproate) or atypical antipsychotic (quetiapine, olanzapine, risperidone, aripiprazole). Bipolar depression → quetiapine, lurasidone, lamotrigine, or lithium. Monitor labs (lithium level/Cr/TSH; valproate LFTs/platelets). Urgent psychiatry if uncertain.

3. ADHD (adults): stimulants (methylphenidate/ amphetamine preparations) with BP/HR monitoring and misuse risk assessment; non-stimulants (atomoxetine, bupropion, guanfacine XR/clonidine XR) when contraindications or misuse risk. Combine with skills coaching.

4. Anxiety disorders: SSRIs/SNRIs first-line; start low and titrate to effect; allow 4–8 wks. Hydroxyzine PRN for short-term relief. Avoid chronic benzodiazepines;

consider brief use (2–4 wks max) in severe panic while initiating SSRI with close follow-up.

5. Psychotic disorders (first episode): urgent psychiatry/ early psychosis program. Start second-generation antipsychotic if needed (aripiprazole, risperidone, olanzapine, quetiapine) at low dose; monitor metabolic profile (weight, BP, A1C, lipids) and EPS. Consider LAI in recurrent non-adherence (specialist-led).

6. Substance use disorders:

7. Alcohol: first-line medications — naltrexone (oral daily or monthly injection) or acamprosate (TID if normal renal); consider disulfiram with supervision. Add counseling; thiamine if heavy use/withdrawal risk.

8. Opioids: buprenorphine-naloxone in primary care (if within scope); check for withdrawal before induction; provide naloxone to all at risk. Extended-release naltrexone is alternative after detox; methadone via specialized clinics.

9. Tobacco: varenicline, bupropion SR, or combination NRT; behavioral support improves quit rates.

10. Stimulants/cannabis: no approved meds; use contingency management, CBT, harm reduction; treat comorbid ADHD/depression appropriately.

C. PROCEDURES

1. Create written safety plans; prescribe naloxone kits; arrange long-acting injectable antipsychotics where indicated (via psychiatry).

2. Coordinate collaborative care (care manager +

consulting psychiatrist) to improve outcomes; set up follow-ups (1–2 wks after starts/changes).

DISPOSITION (DISCHARGE/OBSERVE/ TRANSFER) & RETURN PRECAUTIONS

1. Immediate ED/psychiatry: active suicidal intent/ plan or recent attempt, psychosis with risk/command hallucinations, mania with danger or inability to care for self, severe withdrawal (delirium tremens, seizures), serotonin syndrome, NMS, catatonia, postpartum psychosis.

2. Urgent (24–72 h): new first-episode psychosis without imminent danger, moderate–severe depression with passive SI but no plan, complicated medication starts (e.g., lithium/valproate monitoring), failure of two adequate antidepressant trials.

3. Return immediately for: new/worsening SI/HI, severe agitation or confusion, chest pain/palpitations on stimulants/antipsychotics, rash/fever on lamotrigine (SJS concern).

PEARLS & PITFALLS

1. Always screen for bipolar before starting antidepressants; a history of decreased need for sleep and periods of elevated energy is key.

2. Start low, go slow — but go: titrate to therapeutic doses and treat to remission, not just improvement.

3. Review drug–drug interactions (e.g., SSRIs with

triptans/MAOIs/linezolid; bupropion lowers seizure
threshold; QTc with citalopram/antipsychotics).

4. Avoid long-term benzodiazepines; prefer CBT and
   SSRIs/SNRIs for chronic anxiety.

5. Combine meds + psychotherapy + social supports;
   arrange close follow-up after initiation/changes (1–2
   weeks).

REFERENCES

1. NICE CKS & Guidelines: Depression in adults;
   Bipolar disorder; Generalised anxiety disorder & panic
   disorder; Psychosis and schizophrenia; ADHD (public).
   nice.org.uk / cks.nice.org.uk

2. AAFP. Pharmacologic Treatment of Depression;
   Generalized Anxiety Disorder and Panic Disorder;
   Bipolar Disorders: Evaluation and Treatment; Adult
   ADHD; First-Episode Psychosis; Alcohol & Opioid Use
   Disorders (open articles). aafp.org

3. APA (American Psychiatric Association) guideline
   resources & patient pages (public summaries).
   psychiatry.org

4. NIMH (National Institute of Mental Health) — Illness
   overviews and treatment basics (public). nimh.nih.gov

5. SAMHSA. TIPs and SBIRT tools; Buprenorphine quick
   start guide; Overdose prevention & naloxone (public).
   samhsa.gov

6. VA/DoD Clinical Practice Guidelines (open PDFs):
   Major Depressive Disorder; Management of SUD;

Psychosis (public). healthquality.va.gov

7. WHO mhGAP Intervention Guide — mental, neurological and substance use disorders in non-specialized settings (open). who.int

ALCOHOL USE DISORDER — INCLUDING WITHDRAWAL & INTOXICATION

OVERVIEW & "DON'T MISS"

1. AUD is common and treatable; withdrawal ranges from mild tremor/anxiety → seizures (6–48 h) → delirium tremens (48–96 h).

2. Intoxication can mask trauma, infection, hypoglycemia, or co-ingestions; consider toxic alcohols if high anion/osmolar gap or visual symptoms.

3. DON'T MISS: Wernicke encephalopathy (confusion, ataxia, ophthalmoplegia — triad often incomplete) → give parenteral thiamine immediately; alcohol withdrawal seizures; DTs; hypoglycemia; head injury; GI bleed; pancreatitis; aspiration; suicidal ideation.

HISTORY & EXAM

1. Use brief validated screens: AUDIT-C or single-item screen; quantify typical week and heaviest day; last drink; prior severe withdrawal/ICU; seizures/DTs; comorbidities; pregnancy; meds (benzodiazepines, opioids).

2. Withdrawal symptoms: tremor, anxiety, sweating, tachycardia, insomnia, N/V, hallucinosis; timing vs. last drink. Intoxication: slurred speech, ataxia, nystagmus, altered level — check for injuries.

3. Exam: vitals (tachycardia, HTN, fever), hydration, neuro (tremor, confusion), abdominal tenderness (hepatitis/pancreatitis), signs of chronic liver disease; look for trauma.

4. Risk stratify: CIWA-Ar for symptom severity (primary care: mild ≤10–12), PAWSS for predicting complicated withdrawal; social supports at home.

DIFFERENTIAL DIAGNOSIS (TOP 5)

1. Withdrawal vs. anxious state or stimulant withdrawal.

2. Hypoglycemia, sepsis, meningitis/encephalitis causing agitation/AMS.

3. Head injury/intracranial bleed (especially with anticoagulants).

4. Toxic alcohols (methanol/ethylene glycol) — high gap acidosis, visual loss, flank pain.

5. Hepatic encephalopathy (asterixis, ammonia), pancreatitis, GI bleed.

INVESTIGATIONS (POC/LABS/IMAGING)

1. POC glucose for all; pregnancy test if applicable; alcohol level if management/medico-legal need.

2. Labs as indicated: electrolytes (Na/K/Mg/PO4), creatinine, LFTs, INR, CBC; lipase if pain; VBG/ABG

with anion gap ± osmolar gap if acidosis/suspicion for toxic alcohols.

3. Urine tox (limited utility) and targeted co-ingestions; ECG (QTc, arrhythmias). CT head if trauma/LOC/ anticoagulation or focal neuro deficits.

4. Use CIWA-Ar to guide symptom-triggered therapy when appropriate settings/staffing exist.

MANAGEMENT (NON-PHARM → MEDS → PROCEDURES)

A. NON-PHARMACOLOGIC

1. Safety: monitor in appropriate setting; treat pain/ anxiety; dark, quiet room; supportive counselling & motivational interviewing; harm-reduction and linkage to community supports.

2. Nutrition: thiamine BEFORE glucose when possible; folate and multivitamin; correct fluids/electrolytes (especially Mg, K, PO4).

3. Discharge planning: written plan, follow-up, crisis resources; driving/occupational advice.

B. MEDICATIONS (EXAMPLES; INDIVIDUALIZE, CHECK LOCAL PROTOCOLS)

1. Thiamine: 200–500 mg IV q8–24h for 2–3 days if Wernicke suspected or high risk (malnourished, withdrawal, AMS), then 100 mg PO/IV daily. Give BEFORE glucose when feasible.

2. Withdrawal (benzodiazepines first-line):

3. Symptom-triggered (preferred when staff trained): diazepam 10–20 mg PO/IV q1–2h PRN or lorazepam 2–4 mg PO/IV q1–2h PRN until calm/lightly drowsy; reassess with CIWA-Ar.

4. Fixed-dose (when symptom-triggered not feasible): diazepam 10 mg PO q6h day 1, then taper 3–5 days; or chlordiazepoxide 25–50 mg PO q6h then taper. Use lorazepam in liver disease/elderly.

5. Refractory/severe or ED/ICU: consider phenobarbital protocols; adjuncts like dexmedetomidine/propofol in ICU — specialist care.

6. Adjuncts/alternatives for mild outpatient withdrawal: gabapentin 300 mg TID (taper) ± carbamazepine 200 mg QID (avoid in severe withdrawal/seizure history). Avoid antipsychotics as monotherapy (lower seizure threshold); can add haloperidol for severe agitation with benzodiazepines.

7. Intoxication: airway protection, dextrose if hypoglycemic after thiamine, IV fluids as needed; monitor for trauma/aspiration; avoid 'sobering' meds.

8. Suspected toxic alcohols: fomepizole per protocol, bicarbonate for acidosis, urgent nephrology/poison centre; consider dialysis.

9. Relapse prevention (initiate once withdrawal controlled and patient ready):

10. Naltrexone 50 mg PO daily (or monthly LAI) — contraindicated with opioids and acute hepatitis/liver

failure; check LFTs.

11. Acamprosate 666 mg PO TID (renally cleared; avoid if CrCl <30 mL/min).

12. Disulfiram 250 mg PO daily — consider motivated patients with supervision; counsel on reaction and interactions; not first-line for most.

13. Off-label options (evidence mixed): topiramate, gabapentin — consider if first-line not tolerated/ contraindicated.

C. PROCEDURES

1. Airway management for severe intoxication/DTs; seizure management per ACLS (benzodiazepines first).

2. IV access, cardiac and oximetry monitoring for moderate–severe withdrawal; consider admission pathways; CIWA-Ar monitoring protocol.

DISPOSITION (DISCHARGE/OBSERVE/ TRANSFER) & RETURN PRECAUTIONS

1. Discharge: mild withdrawal controlled, reliable supports, safe housing, clear outpatient plan for meds and follow-up (48–72 h).

2. Observe/admit: CIWA-Ar persistently high (>15–20), history of severe withdrawal/DTs, seizures, significant comorbidity (cirrhosis, COPD, CAD), pregnancy, polysubstance use, unstable vitals, lack of social supports.

3. Transfer/ED: suspected DTs, refractory agitation, seizures, toxic alcohol ingestion, severe head injury, GI bleed, pancreatitis, severe electrolyte derangements.

4. Return immediately for: worsening confusion/agitation, hallucinations, seizures, chest pain/SOB, severe vomiting, melena/hematemesis, vision changes (toxic alcohol).

PEARLS & PITFALLS

1. Always give parenteral thiamine early in at-risk patients; don't wait for labs.

2. Use lorazepam over diazepam in significant hepatic impairment, frailty, or respiratory compromise.

3. Symptom-triggered benzodiazepine dosing reduces total dose and length of stay when staffing allows.

4. Screen for depression, anxiety, PTSD, suicidality; offer harm-reduction and psychosocial supports alongside meds.

5. Arrange hepatitis A/B vaccination and liver disease screening; consider pregnancy testing and contraception counselling where applicable.

REFERENCES

1. NIAAA (National Institute on Alcohol Abuse and Alcoholism). Helping Patients Who Drink Too Much: A Clinician's Guide (update, online). niaaa.nih.gov

2. ASAM. The ASAM Clinical Practice Guideline on Alcohol Withdrawal Management (open executive

summaries). asam.org

3. NICE CKS. Alcohol-use disorders (harmful drinking and alcohol dependence) and Alcohol withdrawal (public). cks.nice.org.uk

4. WHO mhGAP Intervention Guide — management of substance use (alcohol) and withdrawal (open). who. int

5. Emergency Care BC. Alcohol Withdrawal — Clinical Summary (public). emergencycarebc.ca

6. BC Centre on Substance Use (BCCSU). Provincial guidance on AUD medications and withdrawal (public). bccsu.ca

7. Poison Control/TOXBASE/US CDC clinical toxicology pages for toxic alcohols and fomepizole use (public). cdc.gov / local poison centre websites

ALCOHOL USE DISORDER — OFFICE MANAGEMENT

OVERVIEW & "DON'T MISS"

1. Goal: identify unhealthy alcohol use/AUD, manage in primary care with brief interventions, medications, monitoring, and harm-reduction.

2. Use SBIRT framework (Screening, Brief Intervention, Referral to Treatment).

3. DON'T MISS: risk of severe withdrawal (prior DTs/ seizures, heavy daily use, severe comorbidity), suicidality, pregnancy, domestic violence, co-use of sedatives/opioids (overdose risk), acute liver failure, pancreatitis.

HISTORY & EXAM

1. Screening: AUDIT-C (≥3 women/≥4 men positive) → full AUDIT; single-item screen if time-limited.

2. Assess DSM-5 criteria count for severity (mild 2–3, moderate 4–5, severe ≥6).

3. Pattern: typical week/heaviest day, binges, blackouts; last drink; prior quit attempts; withdrawal history;

triggers; goals (cut down vs abstain).

4. Co-use: opioids/benzos/stimulants/cannabis; meds (disulfiram interactions), allergies.

5. Comorbids: depression/anxiety/PTSD, liver disease, pancreatitis, OSA, cardiomyopathy; pregnancy/ contraception.

6. Exam: vitals; tremor; mental state; signs of liver disease (spider naevi, hepatomegaly), neuropathy; injuries.

DIFFERENTIAL DIAGNOSIS (TOP 5)

1. Unhealthy alcohol use without AUD (no impairment/ distress).

2. Sedative-hypnotic use disorder; concurrent opioid use disorder.

3. Primary mood/anxiety disorder vs. substance-induced.

4. Alcohol-related liver disease vs. viral/NAFLD.

5. Wernicke-Korsakoff syndrome vs. other cognitive disorders.

INVESTIGATIONS (POC/LABS/IMAGING)

1. Baseline labs: CBC (MCV, platelets), CMP (AST/ALT, ALP, bilirubin, albumin), GGT; creatinine/eGFR; fasting glucose/A1C; lipids.

2. Viral hepatitis (HBsAg ± anti-HBc, anti-HCV) and HIV based on risk; pregnancy test if applicable.

3. Consider PEth (blood) or EtG/EtS (urine) for monitoring in select cases; not routine for therapeutic

alliance.

4. Liver fibrosis assessment: APRI/FIB-4 or elastography if available; ultrasound if LFTs persistently abnormal or red flags.

5. Before meds: LFTs for naltrexone/disulfiram; renal function for acamprosate; ensure opioid-free before naltrexone.

MANAGEMENT (NON-PHARM → MEDS → PROCEDURES)

A. NON-PHARMACOLOGIC

1. Brief intervention (5–15 min): feedback on risk, explore pros/cons, set a SMART goal, negotiate plan (cut down vs abstain), arrange follow-up.

2. Motivational interviewing: ask-permission → provide information → elicit change talk; use readiness ruler (0–10).

3. Harm-reduction: do not drink and drive; avoid mixing with sedatives/opioids; food/hydration; set alcohol-free days; smaller containers; safer environments.

4. Psychosocial: CBT, mutual-help (AA/SMART Recovery), digital supports; address housing/violence; involve family with consent.

B. MEDICATIONS (FIRST-LINE & ALTERNATIVES; INDIVIDUALIZE)

1. Thiamine: 100 mg PO daily prophylaxis (higher/IV if

malnourished or withdrawal risk). Add multivitamin ± folate.

2. Naltrexone 50 mg PO daily (or monthly XR where available) — start even if still drinking; check LFTs; avoid with opioids or acute hepatitis/liver failure; counsel on reduced heavy-drinking days.

3. Acamprosate 666 mg PO TID — start after abstinent or within 7 days of cessation; renally cleared (333 mg TID if CrCl 30–50; avoid if <30). Best for maintaining abstinence.

4. Disulfiram 250 mg PO daily — only for motivated patients with supervision; counsel on reaction with any alcohol (incl. sauces, cosmetics); baseline and periodic LFTs; contraindicated in severe heart disease, psychosis, pregnancy; avoid in significant liver disease.

5. Off-label options (when first-line unsuitable): topiramate (titrate to 100–300 mg/day; monitor cognition/paresthesias), gabapentin (up to 1800 mg/ day; sedation). SSRIs treat comorbid depression but do not treat AUD.

6. Co-use opioids: provide naloxone kit and counsel on overdose; coordinate OUD treatment if present.

C. PROCEDURES

1. None routine in office; consider point-of-care breathalyzer for feedback. Vaccinate for Hep A/B if not immune; Tdap/influenza/COVID per schedule.

DISPOSITION (DISCHARGE/OBSERVE/ TRANSFER) & RETURN PRECAUTIONS

1. Office-based management appropriate when: mild–moderate AUD, no history of severe withdrawal/DTs, stable housing/supports, no active suicidality, and medically stable.

2. Refer/urgent pathways: history of severe withdrawal/ DTs or withdrawal seizures, CIWA-Ar ≥10–12 with limited supports, severe liver disease (jaundice, INR↑, ascites), pregnancy, polysubstance use with sedatives, unsafe living situation.

3. Follow-up: weekly for 4–6 weeks, then monthly; track days abstinent, heavy-drinking days, cravings, side effects; recheck LFTs 4–12 weeks after starting naltrexone/disulfiram.

4. Return immediately/ED: severe vomiting, confusion, seizures, syncope, melena/hematemesis, chest pain/ SOB, thoughts of self-harm.

PEARLS & PITFALLS

1. Offer medication to ALL with moderate–severe AUD who are open to it — it roughly doubles success versus counselling alone.

2. Starting naltrexone without a period of abstinence is acceptable; focus on reducing heavy-drinking days if abstinence not yet achievable.

3. Supervise disulfiram for effectiveness and safety; stop if transaminases rise significantly.

4. Build a no-shame, iterative plan — relapse is part of recovery; adjust meds/psychosocial supports and continue follow-up.

5. Document goals, consent, and safety-netting at every visit.

REFERENCES

1. NIAAA. Helping Patients Who Drink Too Much: A Clinician's Guide (online). niaaa.nih.gov

2. USPSTF. Unhealthy Alcohol Use in Adolescents and Adults: Screening and Behavioral Counseling Interventions (2018, reaffirmed updates online). uspreventiveservicestaskforce.org

3. NICE CKS. Alcohol-use disorders — identification and management; pharmacological management (public). cks.nice.org.uk

4. BC Centre on Substance Use (BCCSU). Provincial guideline on AUD medications (public). bccsu.ca

5. WHO mhGAP. Management of substance use (alcohol) in non-specialized settings (open). who.int

6. Canadian Centre on Substance Use and Addiction (CCSA). Canada's Guidance on Alcohol and Health (2023). ccsa.ca

7. Emergency Care BC / Public resources on withdrawal risk and referral pathways (public). emergencycarebc. ca

OPIOID USE DISORDER — INCLUDING WITHDRAWAL & INTOXICATION

OVERVIEW & "DON'T MISS"

1. OUD is chronic, relapsing but treatable; MOUD (buprenorphine or methadone) reduces mortality and improves retention.

2. Intoxication triad: miosis + respiratory depression + decreased LOC; co-ingestants (benzos, alcohol) ↑ overdose risk.

3. Withdrawal: not life-threatening but very distressing — begins 6–24 h after short-acting opioids, later for long-acting or methadone.

4. DON'T MISS: apnea/respiratory failure, aspiration, toxic co-ingestions (sedatives, alcohol), severe dehydration/electrolyte derangements, pregnancy (maternal overdose still requires naloxone), precipitated withdrawal with premature buprenorphine dosing.

HISTORY & EXAM

1. Substance history: type (heroin/fentanyl/oxycodone/

methadone), route, amount, last use, prior overdoses/ Naloxone, current MOUD (dose/last dose), co-use (benzos, alcohol, stimulants).

2. Medical/psych: pregnancy, chronic pain, liver/renal disease, QT risk, mental health, suicidality, infectious risks (HIV/HCV).

3. Withdrawal symptoms: anxiety, yawning, lacrimation/ rhinorrhea, piloerection, mydriasis, N/V/D, cramps, myalgias, insomnia. Use COWS to quantify (mild 5–12, mod 13–24, severe ≥25).

4. Exam: vitals, RR, O2 sat, capnography if available, pupils, mental status; look for track marks/skin/ abscesses; chest/abdomen; assess dehydration; consider trauma screen.

DIFFERENTIAL DIAGNOSIS (TOP 5)

1. Sedative-hypnotic intoxication (benzodiazepines, alcohol) ± head injury.

2. Hypoglycemia; sepsis; stroke/ICH; carbon monoxide poisoning.

3. Asthma/COPD exacerbation or pneumonia causing hypoxia/hypercapnia.

4. Clonidine/lofexidine or α-2 agonist toxicity mimicking opioid toxidrome.

5. Serotonin syndrome or anticholinergic toxidrome (opposite pupils/skin findings).

INVESTIGATIONS (POC/LABS/IMAGING)

1. POC glucose for all with AMS; pulse oximetry ± capnography; ECG (QTc if methadone or polypharmacy).

2. Labs (as indicated): BMP (K/Mg), LFTs, CBC, VBG/ABG if hypoventilation, troponin if chest pain, pregnancy test if applicable; CK if prolonged immobilization.

3. Urine drug screens have limited sensitivity for fentanyl/novel opioids; negative screen does not exclude exposure.

4. CXR if aspiration suspected; consider head CT for trauma/anticoagulation or focal deficits.

MANAGEMENT (NON-PHARM → MEDS → PROCEDURES)

A. NON-PHARMACOLOGIC

1. Overdose: airway positioning, rescue breathing, oxygen, bag-valve-mask as needed; call EMS early.

2. Harm reduction: provide take-home naloxone and training; counsel never use alone, test dose, avoid mixing with sedatives/alcohol; consider fentanyl test strips where legal.

3. Linkage: same-day MOUD initiation when possible; arrange follow-up, social work, housing, and infection screening/vaccination (Hep A/B).

B. MEDICATIONS (EXAMPLES; INDIVIDUALIZE; CHECK LOCAL REGULATIONS)

1. Naloxone for suspected overdose:

2. IN 4 mg (one spray) or IM 0.4–2 mg; repeat q2–3 min, titrate to adequate respirations (RR ≥12) rather than full arousal. Consider infusion (≈ two-thirds of effective 'wake-up' dose per hour) for long-acting opioids.

3. Expect re-sedation with methadone/ER opioids; observe longer or use infusion.

4. Buprenorphine-naloxone (first-line MOUD):

5. Standard induction when in moderate withdrawal (COWS ≥8–12): start 2–4 mg SL, reassess q1–2 h to 8–16 mg total day 1; typical day 2 12–24 mg (max per local guidance).

6. To avoid precipitated withdrawal (esp. high-potency fentanyl exposure), use adequate washout/withdrawal before first dose, OR consider low-dose 'micro-induction' while continuing a small amount of full agonist (specialist protocols).

7. Pregnancy: use buprenorphine mono-product; coordinate with obstetrics.

8. Methadone (full agonist MOUD):

9. Initial 20–30 mg once daily (lower in elderly/hepatic/respiratory disease); observe for sedation; avoid >30 mg on day 1 unless specialist/ED monitoring.

10. Titrate cautiously by 5–10 mg every 3–5 days to control cravings/withdrawal; obtain baseline and follow-up ECG if QT risk. Watch CYP interactions (e.g.,

azoles, macrolides).

11. Withdrawal symptom relief (if MOUD deferred or as adjunct):

12. Clonidine 0.1–0.2 mg PO q6–8 h PRN (hold if SBP <100). Lofexidine where available.

13. Adjuncts: ondansetron, loperamide, NSAIDs/ acetaminophen, trazodone/hydroxyzine for sleep/ anxiety, tizanidine/gabapentin PRN (caution sedation).

14. Naltrexone (extended-release): option only after 7–10 days opioid-free; caution overdose risk if stopped — generally not first-line in primary care compared with MOUD.

C. PROCEDURES

1. Airway management for severe intoxication; consider naloxone infusion via IV pump.

2. Point-of-care ultrasound for aspiration/pulmonary edema if trained; incision & drainage of injection-related abscesses when indicated (separate protocols).

DISPOSITION (DISCHARGE/OBSERVE/ TRANSFER) & RETURN PRECAUTIONS

1. Discharge: stable vitals, able to ambulate, no ongoing sedation after observation (longer for methadone/ ER opioids), started on MOUD or expedited referral, take-home naloxone provided.

2. Observe/Admit: repeated naloxone doses or infusion,

polysubstance sedation, aspiration pneumonia, pregnancy, severe comorbidity, suicidal ideation, or lack of safe supports.

3. Return immediately for: increasing sleepiness, slowed breathing, cyanosis, chest pain, severe vomiting, or new confusion; call EMS after naloxone use.

PEARLS & PITFALLS

1. Treat to breathing, not to arousal — excessive naloxone can precipitate severe withdrawal and agitation.

2. Avoid starting buprenorphine too early; confirm objective withdrawal (COWS) or use micro-induction strategies.

3. MOUD is the gold standard — offer to all with OUD; continue during hospitalization and peri-procedurally.

4. Avoid co-prescribing benzodiazepines with opioids; if already co-used, treat OUD but counsel on overdose risk and consider slower inductions.

5. Provide written instructions, community resources, and document follow-up within 24–72 h.

REFERENCES

1. SAMHSA TIP 63. Medications for Opioid Use Disorder (2018+ updates) — public PDF. samhsa.gov

2. ASAM National Practice Guideline for the Treatment of Opioid Use Disorder (2020+ updates; executive summaries open). asam.org

3. BC Centre on Substance Use (BCCSU). Buprenorphine/Naloxone and Methadone Clinical Guidelines (open). bccsu.ca

4. CDC. Opioid Overdose — naloxone guidance, prevention resources. cdc.gov

5. CA Bridge/ACEP resources on ED-initiated buprenorphine (open). bridgetotreatment.org

6. WHO. Guidelines for the psychosocially assisted pharmacological treatment of opioid dependence (public). who.int

7. NICE CKS. Drug misuse management in over 16s — opioid dependence (public). cks.nice.org.uk

8. Emergency Care BC. Opioid Use Disorder, Withdrawal, and Overdose clinical summaries (public). emergencycarebc.ca

ENT / OPHTHALMOLOGY

EAR PAIN — OFFICE/URGENT CARE (OTITIS EXTERNA/MEDIA INCL. FUNGAL, FOREIGN BODY)

OVERVIEW & "DON'T MISS"

1. Common causes: otitis externa (bacterial/fungal), acute otitis media (AOM), otitis media with effusion (OME), barotrauma, Eustachian tube dysfunction, cerumen impaction, foreign body, referred pain (dental/TMJ/pharynx).

2. DON'T MISS: malignant/necrotizing otitis externa (elderly/diabetics, severe pain, granulation tissue), mastoiditis (post-auricular swelling/tenderness, fever), cholesteatoma (retraction pocket/foul otorrhea), perichondritis after piercing, Ramsay Hunt (zoster oticus with facial palsy), temporal bone fracture, sudden sensorineural hearing loss, button battery in canal.

HISTORY & EXAM

1. History: onset/tempo, swimming/water exposure, recent URI, flying/diving, trauma/Q-tip use, contact

with ill persons, foreign body suspicion, diabetes/ immunosuppression, prior ear surgery/tubes.

2. Symptoms: pain character (movement/touch worsens in OE), pruritus (often fungal OE), discharge (color/ odor), hearing change (conductive vs sensorineural), vertigo, tinnitus, fever, trismus.

3. Exam: vitals; pinna/tragus tenderness (OE), auricle erythema (perichondritis). Otoscopy: canal edema/ debris, TM color/position/mobility (pneumatic), perforation; mastoid erythema/tenderness; cranial nerves (facial nerve). Avoid irrigation if perforation suspected.

DIFFERENTIAL DIAGNOSIS (TOP 5)

1. Acute otitis externa (bacterial); fungal OE (otomycosis).

2. Acute otitis media (AOM) vs. otitis media with effusion (OME).

3. Foreign body or cerumen impaction; canal furunculosis.

4. Barotrauma/Eustachian tube dysfunction.

5. Referred otalgia (dental caries/TMJ disorder/ pharyngitis/cervical spine).

INVESTIGATIONS (POC/LABS/IMAGING)

1. Usually clinical. Tympanometry (AOM/OME) and tuning-fork (Weber/Rinne) if hearing change. Swab canal discharge only if severe, recurrent,

post-operative, or not responding to therapy (including suspected fungal).

2. Glucose/ESR/CRP and CT temporal bone if malignant OE suspected; urgent ENT.

3. Audiology for persistent hearing loss, OME ≥3 months, sudden SNHL (urgent).

4. Avoid ear irrigation with suspected TM perforation, tubes, or button battery/vegetable matter foreign bodies.

MANAGEMENT (NON-PHARM → MEDS → PROCEDURES)

A. NON-PHARMACOLOGIC

1. Analgesia is key (acetaminophen/ibuprofen; brief opiate only if severe). Keep ear dry; stop Q-tips. Dry-ear precautions after swimming (ear plugs/shower cap).

2. Aural toilet: gentle suction/debridement if trained; consider ear wick for swollen canal in OE to deliver drops.

3. Education: return precautions; avoid flying/diving until symptoms resolve if barotrauma/OME.

B. MEDICATIONS (EXAMPLES; INDIVIDUALIZE & VERIFY DOSING/CONTRAINDICATIONS)

1. Otitis externa — bacterial:

2. First-line topical drops × 7–10 d: fluoroquinolone

(ofloxacin or ciprofloxacin) ± steroid; or neomycin/
polymyxin B/hydrocortisone ONLY if intact TM and
no neomycin allergy. Use wick if marked edema.
Re-check in 48–72 h if severe.

3. Systemic antibiotics only if extension beyond canal,
    diabetes/immunocompromised with cellulitis, or failed
    topical therapy.

4. Otitis externa — fungal (otomycosis):

5. Meticulous debridement + clotrimazole 1% ear drops
    BID–TID × 7–14 d (or acetic acid 2% QID). Avoid
    steroid-only products; keep ear dry. Consider culture if
    refractory.

6. Malignant/necrotizing OE (elderly/diabetic, severe
    pain, granulation tissue, cranial neuropathy):

7. URGENT ENT/ED; antipseudomonal therapy (often
    IV). Oral ciprofloxacin may be used initially in selected
    stable cases per local protocol but requires specialist
    oversight; obtain imaging and inflammatory markers.

8. AOM (children/adults):

9. Pain control first. Children: consider observation 24–48
    h if mild and age >6 months; otherwise high-dose
    amoxicillin 80–90 mg/kg/day divided BID (max 2 g/
    dose). Penicillin allergy (non-anaphylactic): cefdinir/
    cefuroxime; anaphylaxis: azithromycin (lower efficacy).
    Duration 5–10 d by age/severity.

10. Adults: amoxicillin-clavulanate 875/125 mg BID 5–7
    d if bacterial suspected. TM perforation/otorrhea:
    add topical fluoroquinolone ear drops; avoid

aminoglycosides.

11. OME (no acute infection):

12. No antibiotics. Watchful waiting 3 months; nasal steroids and allergy control if allergic rhinitis; autoinflation. ENT/audiology if persistent, at-risk speech delay, or unilateral adult OME (exclude nasopharyngeal pathology).

13. Perichondritis (piercing/trauma):

14. Cover Pseudomonas & Staph: ciprofloxacin 500 mg BID 7–10 d; admit/IV if abscess or systemic signs; ENT for drainage if fluctuance.

15. Ramsay Hunt (herpes zoster oticus) with facial palsy:

16. Start valacyclovir 1 g TID (or acyclovir 800 mg five-times daily) + prednisone ~60 mg daily then taper over 7–10 d within 72 h; eye protection/lubrication and urgent ENT/ophthalmology.

17. Barotrauma/ET dysfunction:

18. Oral/topical nasal decongestants (short course), nasal steroid for allergic rhinitis, auto-insufflation; avoid flying/diving until improved.

19. Cerumen impaction:

20. Cerumenolytics (carbamide peroxide/mineral oil) then irrigation/manual removal if no perforation/tubes/active infection.

21. Foreign body (see Procedures).

C. PROCEDURES

1. Foreign body removal: visualize fully; use right-angle

hook/alligator forceps/suction. Irrigation acceptable for small smooth objects only if intact TM and NOT organic matter (beans), NOT button batteries, and NOT expandable materials.

2. Button battery/magnet in ear canal: URGENT removal (preferably ENT). Do NOT instill drops until type confirmed; document time in canal.

3. Live insect: kill with mineral oil or 2% lidocaine before removal.

4. Post-removal canal abrasion: consider topical antibiotic/steroid drops × 3–5 d; tetanus update if laceration.

DISPOSITION (DISCHARGE/OBSERVE/ TRANSFER) & RETURN PRECAUTIONS

1. ED/Immediate: suspected malignant OE, mastoiditis (post-auricular swelling/tenderness + fever), severe otitis with cranial neuropathy, facial paralysis, toxic patient, temporal bone fracture, button battery in canal, meningitis signs, sudden sensorineural hearing loss.

2. Urgent ENT (24–72 h): refractory OE/AOM, suspected cholesteatoma, persistent unilateral adult OME, recurrent AOM, severe canal edema needing wick, perichondritis with abscess, TM perforation not healing in 6–8 wks, significant hearing loss.

3. Return immediately for: worsening pain/swelling/fever, spreading redness, vertigo, severe headache, mastoid pain, new facial weakness, or persistent otorrhea.

PEARLS & PITFALLS

1. Avoid aminoglycoside ear drops if TM not clearly intact or if tympanostomy tubes present — risk of ototoxicity; use fluoroquinolone drops instead.

2. Pain with pinna/tragus movement points to otitis externa; middle-ear disease less tender to external manipulation.

3. Granulation tissue at bony-cartilaginous junction in diabetics = malignant OE until proven otherwise.

4. Do not irrigate if perforation/tubes present or if organic material/button battery suspected.

5. Adults with unilateral persistent OME need nasopharyngeal evaluation to exclude mass.

REFERENCES

1. NICE CKS. Otitis externa; Otitis media – acute; Otitis media with effusion; Foreign body in ear (public). cks. nice.org.uk

2. AAFP. Otitis Externa: A Practical Guide to Treatment and Prevention; Diagnosis and Treatment of Otitis Media; Cerumen Impaction (open articles). aafp.org

3. CDC. Clinical overviews: Acute Otitis Media; Swimmer's Ear; Shingles (Ramsay Hunt) (public). cdc. gov

4. ENT UK / Patient.info. Perichondritis of the Pinna; Ear Foreign Bodies (public). entuk.org / patient.info

5. Merck Manual Professional. Malignant External Otitis; Barotrauma of the Ear (open). merckmanuals.com

6. Royal Children's Hospital (Melbourne). Clinical Guidelines: Otitis media; Otitis externa; Foreign bodies in the ear (open). rch.org.au

RED EYE IN FAMILY PRACTICE

OVERVIEW & "DON'T MISS"

1. Assess visual acuity FIRST; check pupils, EOMs, and use fluorescein with cobalt blue if available.

2. Red flags → same-day ophthalmology/ED: decreased vision, severe pain, photophobia, corneal opacity/ ulcer, ciliary flush, irregular pupil, hypopyon/hyphema, proptosis, fever with painful EOM (orbital cellulitis), contact-lens wearer with pain/photophobia, trauma/ foreign body, chemical injury.

3. DON'T MISS: acute angle-closure glaucoma, infectious keratitis (esp. contact lens–related), uveitis/ iritis, scleritis, endophthalmitis, orbital cellulitis.

HISTORY & EXAM

1. Onset/tempo (sudden vs gradual), pain vs itch, photophobia, discharge (watery vs purulent vs stringy), contact lens use/sleeping in lenses, trauma/foreign body/grinding, UV/welding exposure, sick contacts, systemic disease (autoimmune), HSV history.

2. Examine: VA each eye (pinhole), pupils (APD), pattern (diffuse vs sectoral vs ciliary flush), lid/lash/

margins, preauricular nodes, cornea clarity/defects (fluorescein), anterior chamber depth/cells/flare if light available, IOP if trained/equipment.

3. Differentiate: conjunctivitis (diffuse injection, minimal pain, normal vision), keratitis/corneal abrasion (focal defect/opacity, photophobia), uveitis (consensual photophobia, small irregular pupil, ciliary flush), scleritis (deep boring pain, violaceous hue), angle-closure (mid-dilated fixed pupil, halos, headache/N/V).

DIFFERENTIAL DIAGNOSIS (TOP 5)

1. Viral conjunctivitis (adenovirus): watery discharge, preauricular nodes, often bilateral sequentially.

2. Bacterial conjunctivitis: purulent discharge, lids stuck in AM; hyperacute (gonococcal) is copious purulent with rapid progression.

3. Allergic conjunctivitis: intense itch, stringy discharge, papillae; seasonal/perennial.

4. Corneal abrasion/foreign body/UV keratitis: severe pain/photophobia; fluorescein uptake; NO contact lenses until healed.

5. Serious causes: infectious keratitis (esp. contact lens Pseudomonas), anterior uveitis/iritis, scleritis, acute angle-closure glaucoma, orbital cellulitis.

INVESTIGATIONS (POC/LABS/IMAGING)

1. Visual acuity (document), fluorescein staining/Seidel

test for leak if trauma, lid eversion for FB.

2. Corneal/culture swab if corneal ulcer/keratitis suspected, hyperacute conjunctivitis, neonatal disease, or refractory cases.

3. IOP measurement if angle-closure suspected and you're trained/equipped; do NOT delay referral.

4. CT orbits/sinuses with contrast if orbital cellulitis suspected (painful EOMs, proptosis, fever, decreased vision).

5. pH testing and irrigation for chemical exposures until 7.0–7.5 (see below).

MANAGEMENT (NON-PHARM → MEDS → PROCEDURES)

A. NON-PHARMACOLOGIC

1. Remove contact lenses; discard current pair; no lens wear until asymptomatic + off antibiotics for 24–48 h.

2. Chemical injury: immediate copious irrigation (normal saline/water) for ≥15–30 min; check pH and continue until 7.0–7.5; evert lids and remove particles; urgent ophthalmology.

3. Cold compresses/lubricants for viral/allergic conjunctivitis; strict hand hygiene; avoid sharing towels; school/daycare exclusion per local policy if significant discharge.

4. Eye protection for UV/welding; avoid rubbing.

B. MEDICATIONS (EXAMPLES; INDIVIDUALIZE &

CHECK LOCAL FORMULARIES/RENAL DOSING)

1. Viral conjunctivitis: supportive only (artificial tears, cool compresses). Topical antibiotics are not required. Consider povidone-iodine in some protocols (specialist-led).

2. Bacterial conjunctivitis (uncomplicated, non–contact lens): trimethoprim-polymyxin B drops q6h or erythromycin ointment q6h × 5–7 d.

3. Contact lens wearers or corneal abrasion with lens use: antipseudomonal fluoroquinolone (ciprofloxacin/ofloxacin/moxifloxacin drops) q2–4h while awake then taper per response; urgent follow-up in 24 h.

4. Allergic conjunctivitis: topical antihistamine/mast-cell stabilizer (e.g., olopatadine) once/twice daily; oral antihistamines if needed; brief low-potency topical steroid ONLY under ophthalmology.

5. Corneal abrasion (non-lens): erythromycin ointment q6h 2–3 d; oral analgesia; consider short-course cyclopentolate for severe photophobia. Do NOT patch the eye. Do NOT prescribe topical anesthetics for home use.

6. Suspected herpetic keratitis (dendrites): avoid steroids; start oral antivirals (acyclovir 400 mg 5×/day or valacyclovir 500 mg TID) and urgent ophthalmology.

7. Anterior uveitis: cycloplegic (cyclopentolate 1% BID–TID) and URGENT ophthalmology for steroid initiation/IOP monitoring.

8. Acute angle-closure glaucoma: EMERGENT

ophthalmology; if within scope while arranging transfer — acetazolamide 500 mg PO/IV then 250 mg q6h, topical timolol 0.5%, apraclonidine 1%, and pilocarpine 1–2% once IOP begins to fall. Analgesia/antiemetic.

9. Orbital cellulitis: immediate ED/IV antibiotics; avoid outpatient management.

C. PROCEDURES

1. Foreign body removal with irrigation/cotton swab after topical anesthetic; avoid metallic drilling in office unless trained.

2. Fluorescein staining + cobalt blue exam; lid eversion to inspect tarsal plate; remove rust ring only if skilled and follow-up assured.

DISPOSITION (DISCHARGE/OBSERVE/ TRANSFER) & RETURN PRECAUTIONS

1. ED/Immediate ophthalmology: decreased vision, severe pain/photophobia, corneal ulcer/opacity, chemical burn, penetrating injury, acute angle-closure, herpetic keratitis, orbital cellulitis.

2. Urgent (24 h) ophthalmology: contact lens–related red eye, persistent abrasion, suspected uveitis, scleritis, hyperacute gonococcal conjunctivitis.

3. Routine follow-up (48–72 h): uncomplicated bacterial/ allergic conjunctivitis; sooner if symptoms worsen.

4. Return immediately for: worsening pain, vision changes, photophobia, swelling, fever, inability to open

eye, or no improvement within 24–48 h.

PEARLS & PITFALLS

1. Document visual acuity before any drops — it's your 'vital sign' for the eye.

2. Contact lens + pain/photophobia = corneal ulcer until proven otherwise — use antipseudomonal coverage and urgent review.

3. Do NOT give topical anesthetic to take home; corneal toxicity and delayed healing can result.

4. Avoid topical steroids unless directed by ophthalmology (worsen HSV keratitis and some infections).

5. Subconjunctival hemorrhage is benign; check BP/anticoagulants; reassure and avoid unnecessary antibiotics.

REFERENCES

1. AAFP. Diagnosis and Management of Red Eye in Primary Care; Evaluation of the Painful Eye (open articles). aafp.org

2. American Academy of Ophthalmology (AAO) public pages: Conjunctivitis, Corneal Abrasion, Uveitis, Keratitis, Angle-Closure Glaucoma, Chemical Injuries. aao.org/eye-health

3. Royal College of Emergency Medicine Learning / Patient.info public resources on red eye and ocular emergencies (open). rcemlearning.co.uk / patient.info

4. NICE CKS. Conjunctivitis (infective/allergic), Red eye, Corneal abrasion (public). cks.nice.org.uk

5. CDC. Gonococcal conjunctivitis; Herpes zoster ophthalmicus — clinical overviews (public). cdc.gov

6. Emergency Care BC. Painful Red Eye; Chemical Eye Injury — clinical summaries (public). emergencycarebc.ca

PHARMACOLOGY / SAFETY

COMMON DRUG INTERACTIONS IN FAMILY MEDICINE

OVERVIEW & "DON'T MISS"

1. Interactions are predictable (PK: CYP/P-gp, renal; PD: additive effects) — many are preventable with checks and monitoring.

2. High-risk flags: anticoagulants/antiplatelets, antiarrhythmics/QT-prolongers, insulin/sulfonylureas, opioids/benzodiazepines, digoxin, lithium, methotrexate, theophylline, immunosuppressants.

3. DON'T MISS outcomes: life-threatening bleeding, torsades de pointes, serotonin syndrome, hyperkalemia/AKI (triple whammy), hypoglycemia, respiratory depression, myopathy/rhabdomyolysis, lithium/digoxin toxicity.

HISTORY & EXAM

1. 'Brown-bag' ALL meds (Rx/OTC/herbals) + alcohol/cannabis; ask about grapefruit/tonics and supplements (St. John's wort, ginkgo, ginseng).

2. Review renal/hepatic function, falls risk, QT history,

and prior ADEs; check pregnancy plans.

3. Look for toxicity signs: bleeding/bruising, confusion, tremor, N/V/D, arrhythmias/syncope, myalgias/ weakness.

DIFFERENTIAL DIAGNOSIS (TOP 5)

1. Adverse drug event from interaction vs. disease progression.

2. Serotonin syndrome vs. NMS vs. anticholinergic toxidrome.

3. Torsades/QT-mediated syncope vs. vasovagal/ orthostatic.

4. Warfarin over-/under-anticoagulation vs. other bleeding disorders.

5. AKI from 'triple whammy' vs. prerenal dehydration/ sepsis.

INVESTIGATIONS (POC/LABS/IMAGING)

1. Targeted monitoring: INR (warfarin) within 3–5 days of interacting drug; K^+/Cr in 3–7 days with ACEi/ARB + K-sparing or 'triple whammy' (ACEi/ARB + diuretic + NSAID); digoxin/lithium levels with symptoms or regimen changes.

2. ECG/QTc when adding QT-prolongers or macrolides/ fluoroquinolones; CK if statin myalgia, LFTs with azoles/macrolides + statins.

3. Use an interaction checker plus provincial monographs; document plan and monitoring intervals.

MANAGEMENT (NON-PHARM → MEDS → PROCEDURES)

A. NON-PHARMACOLOGIC

1. Avoid the combo if a safer option exists; choose agents with fewer interactions (e.g., cephalexin instead of TMP-SMX with warfarin when appropriate).
2. Educate patients to report new OTC/herbals/ supplements and to bring all meds to visits; flag grapefruit interactions.
3. Schedule labs/ECG proactively when initiating known interacting pairs; deprescribe when risks outweigh benefits.

B. COMMON HIGH-YIELD INTERACTIONS (EXAMPLES; NOT EXHAUSTIVE)

Anticoagulants/antiplatelets:

1. Warfarin + TMP-SMX/metronidazole/fluconazole/ amiodarone/clarithromycin → ↑INR/bleeding — use alternatives, lower warfarin dose, and monitor INR closely.
2. Warfarin/DOACs + NSAIDs/SSRI/SNRI → ↑GI bleed — add PPI if necessary, prefer acetaminophen (≤2–3 g/day with warfarin).
3. DOACs (apixaban/rivaroxaban) + strong CYP3A4/P-gp inhibitors (ketoconazole, ritonavir, clarithromycin) → ↑levels; strong inducers (carbamazepine, phenytoin, rifampin, St. John's wort) → ↓levels — avoid or adjust

per label.

Cardiac/QT:

1. Macrolides/fluoroquinolones + antipsychotics/TCAs/ methadone/antiarrhythmics → QT prolongation/ torsades — check baseline QTc, avoid combos if possible.

2. Amiodarone + warfarin/digoxin/statins (simvastatin) → ↑toxicity — reduce doses, monitor INR/digoxin level; limit simvastatin to ≤20 mg (or switch statin).

Lipids:

1. Simvastatin/atorvastatin + strong CYP3A4 inhibitors (clarithromycin, itraconazole, HIV protease inhibitors) or grapefruit → myopathy/rhabdo — hold statin or switch to pravastatin/rosuvastatin; avoid grapefruit.

Electrolytes/renal ('triple whammy'):

1. ACEi/ARB + diuretic + NSAID → AKI/hyperkalemia — avoid; if necessary, hydrate and check Cr/K^+ within 3–7 days.

2. ACEi/ARB + spironolactone/K^+ supplements/ trimethoprim → hyperkalemia — monitor K^+ closely; consider alternatives (e.g., nitrofurantoin instead of TMP for cystitis).

Endocrine/diabetes/thyroid:

1. Sulfonylureas/insulin + quinolones or TMP-SMX → hypoglycemia — monitor and adjust; counsel driving risk.

2. Levothyroxine + calcium/iron/PPIs → ↓absorption — separate by ≥4 hours; recheck TSH.

3. SGLT2 inhibitors + loop diuretics → volume depletion — consider dose adjustment and sick-day rules.

CNS/respiratory:

1. Opioids + benzodiazepines/other sedatives/alcohol → respiratory depression — avoid co-prescribing; provide naloxone.

2. Tramadol + SSRIs/SNRIs/MAOI/linezolid → serotonin syndrome/seizures — avoid; choose non-serotonergic analgesics.

Psych:

1. SSRIs/SNRIs + NSAIDs/anticoagulants → ↑bleeding — consider PPI protection; monitor.

2. Paroxetine/fluoxetine (strong CYP2D6 inhibitors) + tamoxifen → ↓endoxifen (reduced efficacy) — switch to sertraline/citalopram/venlafaxine.

Infectious disease:

1. Clarithromycin (CYP3A4 inhibitor) + calcium-channel blockers (amlodipine) → hypotension — prefer azithromycin; monitor BP.

2. Doxycycline/fluoroquinolones + iron/calcium/antacids → ↓absorption — separate by hours.

GI/Rheum/Heme:

1. Methotrexate (low-dose) + TMP-SMX/trimethoprim → marrow suppression; + NSAIDs → ↑toxicity — avoid;

use folate; monitor CBC/Cr.

2. Allopurinol + azathioprine/6-MP → severe myelosuppression — contraindicated without drastic azathioprine dose reduction and specialist oversight.

Women's health:

1. Combined hormonal contraception + enzyme inducers (rifampin, carbamazepine, phenytoin, St. John's wort) → contraceptive failure — use non-interacting method (IUD, DMPA) or backup.

2. PDE-5 inhibitors + nitrates → profound hypotension — absolute contraindication; caution with α-blockers (separate dosing/monitor BP).

Other:

1. Digoxin + amiodarone/verapamil/macrolides → ↑digoxin — reduce dose and monitor level.

2. Alcohol + metronidazole → disulfiram-like reaction (controversial but counsel avoidance); alcohol + sedatives → additive CNS depression.

C. PROCEDURES

1. Create EMR interaction alerts for the 'big five': anticoagulants, QT-prolongers, opioids/benzos, lithium/digoxin, methotrexate.

2. Use pharmacy collaboration for complex regimens; provide patient handouts on grapefruit, OTC NSAIDs, and supplements.

DISPOSITION (DISCHARGE/OBSERVE/ TRANSFER) & RETURN PRECAUTIONS

1. Discharge with written monitoring plan (which lab, when, action thresholds) and clear symptom triggers (bleeding, syncope, palpitations, muscle pain, confusion).

2. Observe/urgent: marked INR changes, new syncope/ QT prolongation, symptomatic hyperkalemia, serotonin syndrome, severe hypoglycemia, opioid/benzo oversedation.

3. ED/Transfer: torsades/unstable arrhythmia, major bleed, severe myopathy/rhabdomyolysis, lithium/ digoxin toxicity, anaphylaxis.

PEARLS & PITFALLS

1. Start low/go slow and re-check after any change; interactions often appear within days.

2. If you must combine, document rationale and monitoring steps; prefer shorter courses and lowest effective doses.

3. Remember herbals and foods (St. John's wort, grapefruit, vitamin K foods for warfarin).

4. Renal impairment magnifies many interactions — adjust doses and monitoring.

5. When in doubt, check twice (drug checker + product monograph) and phone the pharmacist.

REFERENCES

1. FDA. Drug Development and Drug Interactions: Table of Substrates, Inhibitors and Inducers (public). fda.gov

2. Specialist Pharmacy Service (UK NHS). Medicines Interactions resources — macrolides/statins/QT, warfarin interactions, CYP guidance (public). sps.nhs.uk

3. CredibleMeds®. QTDrugs Lists and clinical resources (patient/clinician) — public access. crediblemeds.org

4. Thrombosis Canada. Practical warfarin guide & drug interactions (open access). thrombosiscanada.ca

5. NICE CKS / BNFC open pages. Warfarin, DOACs, Tamoxifen interactions, Oral contraception with enzyme inducers (public). cks.nice.org.uk

6. Health Canada. Drug Product Database — product monographs (public). canada.ca

7. bpacnz (Best Practice Advocacy Centre New Zealand). Common interactions in primary care articles (open). bpac.org.nz

MEDICATIONS IN RENAL IMPAIRMENT — DOSING & SAFETY BY CKD STAGE (FAMILY MEDICINE OFFICE)

OVERVIEW & "DON'T MISS"

1. Kidney dysfunction alters drug clearance, distribution, and response. Use kidney-safe choices, adjust doses/ intervals, and monitor.

2. Staging (KDIGO): G1 ≥90, G2 60–89, G3a 45–59, G3b 30–44, G4 15–29, G5 <15 mL/min/1.73 m²; 'D' for dialysis. Albuminuria (A1–A3) modifies risk.

3. Use the right estimator: many labels use creatinine clearance (CrCl, Cockcroft–Gault). When label specifies CrCl (e.g., many DOACs), calculate Cockcroft–Gault; do not substitute eGFR unless label allows.

4. DON'T MISS: hyperkalemia (ACEi/ARB/K-sparing/ TMP), lactic acidosis (metformin + AKI/hypoxia), bleeding on DOACs/warfarin with renal decline, opioid/ gabapentinoid over-sedation, digoxin/lithium toxicity,

contrast-associated AKI.

HISTORY & EXAM

1. Medication inventory (Rx/OTC/herbals), sick-day use, recent dehydration/illness, contrast exposure, adherence barriers, and goals of care.

2. Symptoms of drug toxicity: confusion/somnolence, ataxia, tremor, pruritus, N/V, anorexia/weight loss, edema, bleeding/bruising, arrhythmias, cramps.

3. Exam: vitals incl. weight, volume status; edema; uremic signs; neuropathy/myoclonus; skin excoriations; review dialysis schedule if applicable.

DIFFERENTIAL DIAGNOSIS (TOP 5)

1. True AKI vs. pseudo-worsening creatinine (e.g., TMP/ CMV antivirals blocking secretion).

2. Medication toxicity vs. uremic symptoms from CKD progression.

3. Electrolyte-induced arrhythmia/syncope vs. cardiogenic causes.

4. Drug–drug interactions (e.g., macrolide + statin; amiodarone + warfarin/digoxin).

5. Nonadherence or incorrect dosing frequency vs. renal impairment effects.

INVESTIGATIONS (POC/LABS/IMAGING)

1. Baseline & monitoring: BMP (Cr/eGFR, K^+, HCO_3^-), Mg, PO_4; CBC; urinalysis/albumin-creatinine ratio;

weight/BP; ECG if K⁺ abnormal/QT risks.

2. Before/after high-risk changes: check K^+/Cr 1–2 weeks after ACEi/ARB/MRA/TMP start or dose increase; sooner if frail/advanced CKD.

3. Calculate CrCl (Cockcroft–Gault) when labels require it; track trends and dose to current kidney function.

4. If contrast needed: follow local protocols (hydration; avoid nephrotoxic co-meds; use macrocyclic gadolinium in G4–G5 if MRI essential).

MANAGEMENT (NON-PHARM → MEDS → PROCEDURES)

A. NON-PHARMACOLOGIC

1. 'SADMANS' sick-day list: hold during dehydrating illness — Sulfonylureas, ACEi, Diuretics, Metformin, ARBs, NSAIDs, SGLT2 inhibitors; restart when eating/drinking normally and renal function stable.

2. Avoid magnesium/aluminum-containing laxatives/antacids; use PEG/senna and calcium-based binders only if indicated.

3. Hydration counselling; blood pressure, diabetes, and proteinuria control; vaccination (Hep B, influenza, pneumococcal).

B. MEDICATIONS (EXAMPLES; VERIFY LABELS/RENAL TABLES — INDIVIDUALIZE)

1. Analgesics: avoid NSAIDs in G4–G5; use

acetaminophen. Opioids: avoid morphine/codeine in advanced CKD; prefer fentanyl or carefully titrated hydromorphone; reduce tramadol dose/interval.

2. Diabetes: metformin — avoid initiate or stop if eGFR <30; reduce dose and monitor 30–44; hold for contrast/AKI. SGLT2 — benefits in CKD; initiation thresholds per label. DPP-4: sitagliptin/saxagliptin require renal dosing; linagliptin no adjustment. GLP-1 RA: most do not require renal adjustment (avoid exenatide in low eGFR). Insulin requirements ↓ as GFR falls — monitor closely.

3. Cardio/HTN: ACEi/ARB/MRA — check K⁺/Cr 1–2 weeks after changes; acceptable creatinine rise ≤30% from baseline. Thiazides lose efficacy at low GFR; chlorthalidone may work to ~30; use loops G4–G5. Digoxin — reduce dose and monitor level (aim 0.5–0.9 ng/mL).

4. Anticoagulation: dose DOACs by Cockcroft–Gault CrCl per label; warfarin if mechanical valve or severe mitral stenosis. Apixaban often preferred in advanced CKD; involve thrombosis/nephrology for G5/dialysis.

5. Anti-infectives: adjust penicillins/cephalosporins/ fluoroquinolones/acyclovir/vancomycin; avoid aminoglycosides outpatient; nitrofurantoin generally avoid if eGFR <30; TMP-SMX raises K⁺ and SCr — caution with ACEi/ARB/MRA.

6. Neuro/psych: gabapentin/pregabalin — reduce dose markedly; baclofen — avoid or extreme caution (neurotoxicity). Lithium — avoid in moderate-severe

CKD; if used, close level/renal monitoring. SSRIs generally safe; avoid high-dose citalopram (QT).

7. Gout: allopurinol — start low (e.g., 50–100 mg/day) and titrate to urate <360 μmol/L (<6 mg/dL); watch for rash/HLA-B*58:01 in high-risk groups. Febuxostat consider CV risk. Colchicine — reduce dose/interval; avoid with strong CYP3A4/P-gp inhibitors in CKD.

8. GI: PPIs do not need renal dosing but long-term risks; H2 blockers (ranitidine obsolete) — famotidine needs renal adjustment. Laxatives: avoid Mg/phosphate salts; use PEG/senna/docusate.

9. Endocrine: levothyroxine — no renal adjustment; consider lower calcitriol thresholds in G5; avoid alendronate if eGFR <35 (per label); prefer denosumab (monitor hypocalcemia).

10. Respiratory: DOSE adjust oseltamivir; avoid high-dose morphine for dyspnea in CKD; theophylline narrow TI.

11. Derm/others: methotrexate low-dose — avoid if eGFR <30; monitor CBC/Cr; all topical meds OK; avoid high cumulative aluminum exposure.

C. PROCEDURES

1. Contrast studies: weigh risk/benefit; hydrate; withhold nephrotoxins per protocol; for gadolinium in G4–G5 use group II (macrocyclic) agents if essential.

2. Hemodialysis considerations: dose after HD for dialyzable drugs; check renal tables for dialyzability (e.g., give post-HD for many antibiotics, gabapentin). Coordinate with dialysis unit.

DISPOSITION (DISCHARGE/OBSERVE/ TRANSFER) & RETURN PRECAUTIONS

1. Discharge with written plan: targets, doses, hold parameters, and lab schedule (e.g., K^+/Cr 1–2 weeks after changes; ACR q3–6 mo).

2. Urgent review/ED: K^+ ≥6.0 mmol/L or rising, symptomatic uremia, severe acidosis, pulmonary edema, major bleed on anticoagulant, opioid/sedative toxicity, lithium/digoxin toxicity.

3. Return urgently for: vomiting/diarrhea with poor intake (hold SADMANS), weakness/palpitations, confusion/ somnolence, bruising/bleeding.

PEARLS & PITFALLS

1. Dose by CURRENT kidney function; reassess after any acute illness — many 'AKIs' are medication-related and reversible.

2. For CrCl-based labels (e.g., DOACs), use Cockcroft– Gault (actual body weight unless product specifies otherwise).

3. Watch for drugs that raise creatinine without lowering GFR (TMP, cobicistat) — interpret trends clinically.

4. Start low, go slow — but monitor: set dates for K^+/ Cr checks and document acceptable thresholds and actions.

5. When in doubt, use a reputable renal dosing table and call your pharmacist/nephrologist.

REFERENCES

1. KDIGO 2024. Clinical Practice Guideline for the Evaluation and Management of Chronic Kidney Disease — executive summaries and quick reference (open). kdigo.org

2. NICE. Chronic kidney disease: assessment and management — guideline & prescribing considerations (open). nice.org.uk

3. BC Renal. Renal Dosage Adjustment: Common Medications & Dialyzability charts (public PDFs). bcrenal.ca

4. Thrombosis Canada. DOAC Dosing in Atrial Fibrillation & VTE — renal adjustment tables (open). thrombosiscanada.ca

5. NIDDK (NIH). Medicine Safety in CKD — patient/ clinician resources (public). niddk.nih.gov

6. Diabetes Canada. 'SADMANS' Sick-day Medication List — patient handouts (public). diabetes.ca

7. American College of Radiology. Manual on Contrast Media — risk mitigation in CKD (public). acr.org

8. Merck Manual Professional. Chronic Kidney Disease: Drug Dosing and Considerations (open). merckmanuals.com

GENERAL PREVENTION & PUBLIC HEALTH

CANCER SCREENING — BREAST • CERVIX • COLORECTAL • LUNG (ELIGIBLE)

OVERVIEW & "DON'T MISS"

1. Screening = for asymptomatic people; any red-flag symptoms need diagnostic work-up, not screening.

2. Use shared decision-making and follow provincial program criteria (invitation ages/tests may vary).

3. DON'T MISS red flags: new breast lump/skin change, abnormal uterine bleeding or post-coital bleeding, rectal bleeding/iron-deficiency anemia/changed bowels, hemoptysis/unexplained weight loss — investigate urgently.

HISTORY & EXAM

1. Personal risk: prior cancers or polyps, chest radiation, immunosuppression, chronic inflammatory bowel disease; smoking pack-years; obstetric/gynecologic history.

2. Family history: ≥1 first-degree relative with breast/

ovarian/colorectal/lung (age at dx, number affected).

3. Social determinants: access barriers, language, cultural safety; ensure informed consent and privacy.

4. Exam only if symptomatic; otherwise routine vitals and BP.

DIFFERENTIAL DIAGNOSIS (TOP 5)

1. Breast: benign cyst/fibroadenoma; mastitis/abscess; fat necrosis; dermatologic lesions.

2. Cervix: cervicitis, benign polyps, pregnancy-related bleeding, endometrial causes of AUB.

3. Colorectal: hemorrhoids, fissure, IBS, diverticular disease, IBD.

4. Lung: infection, COPD/asthma exacerbation, heart failure, PE (if SOB/hemoptysis).

5. Always consider iron-deficiency anemia, unintentional weight loss, or progressive symptoms as red flags.

INVESTIGATIONS (POC/LABS/IMAGING)

1. Breast (average risk): organized programs commonly invite ages 50–74 for mammography q2–3y; ages 40–49 — individual decision after discussing benefits/harms; follow provincial criteria. Diagnostic mammogram/US if symptomatic.

2. Cervix: screening starts age 21–25 (province-specific) and continues to 65–70. Many programs still use Pap q3y; several transitioning to primary HPV testing q5y. Follow your provincial program.

3. Colorectal (average risk): FIT every 1–2y (most provinces 50–74). Some guidelines strongly recommend 60–74 with individualized decisions 50–59; follow provincial invitation (e.g., SK 50–74). Positive FIT → colonoscopy.

4. Lung (eligible high-risk): low-dose CT (LDCT) annually for adults 55–74 with ≥30 pack-years who currently smoke or quit <15 years; typically up to 3 consecutive annual screens in programs with appropriate expertise.

MANAGEMENT (NON-PHARM → MEDS → PROCEDURES)

A. NON-PHARMACOLOGIC

1. Shared decision-making aids (absolute benefits/ harms), culturally safe counselling, address access barriers, arrange interpreters as needed.

2. Risk reduction: tobacco cessation, HPV vaccination per NACI, physical activity, healthy weight, alcohol moderation, diet rich in fiber/vegetables, sun safety.

B. MEDICATIONS

1. None for screening. (Chemoprevention for high-risk breast cancer is outside scope; refer to specialist/ high-risk clinic when indicated.)

C. PROCEDURES

1. Order program-preferred tests: screening mammography; cervical Pap or HPV test; FIT kits;

LDCT through lung screening program (pre-test eligibility verification).

2. Abnormal results: follow program algorithms (e.g., BI-RADS pathways; ASC-US/LSIL/HPV+ colposcopy; FIT+ colonoscopy within target timelines; LDCT Lung-RADS management).

3. High-risk pathways: refer to genetics/high-risk breast clinic (e.g., BRCA carriers), IBD colonoscopic surveillance, or pulmonary nodule clinics per findings.

DISPOSITION (DISCHARGE/OBSERVE/ TRANSFER) & RETURN PRECAUTIONS

1. Discharge with scheduled screening intervals and clear follow-up plan; document shared decision-making and test chosen/refused.

2. Expedite diagnostic work-up (not screening) for any red-flag symptoms listed on Page 1.

3. Return urgently for: new palpable breast mass/ skin changes; post-coital bleeding or heavy AUB; persistent rectal bleeding/black stools; hemoptysis or unexplained weight loss/night sweats.

PEARLS & PITFALLS

1. Screening is for asymptomatic patients — do not delay diagnostics while arranging screening.

2. Use program kits (FIT) and approved imaging sites to ensure quality and tracking.

3. Document smoking pack-years precisely when

assessing lung eligibility; reassess if quit date changes.

4. For cervical screening, primary HPV testing (where implemented) detects disease earlier with longer intervals than cytology — align with provincial transition timelines.

5. In Saskatchewan: organized programs run for breast, cervical, and colorectal screening; check provincial website for enrolment and intervals.

REFERENCES

1. Canadian Task Force on Preventive Health Care (CTFPHC) — Breast cancer screening (2018; 2024 draft update): canadiantaskforce.ca

2. CTFPHC — Colorectal cancer screening clinician summary/tools (current web pages): canadiantaskforce.ca

3. CTFPHC — Lung cancer screening recommendation (adults 55–74, ≥30 pack-years, quit <15): canadiantaskforce.ca

4. Canadian Partnership Against Cancer — Provincial cervical screening guidance & program transition to HPV testing (2023–2024 environmental scan): partnershipagainstcancer.ca

5. BC Guidelines — Cervical Cancer Prevention and Screening (updated 2025); other program pages (public): bcguidelines.gov.bc.ca

6. Public Health Agency of Canada / Government of

Canada — Cancer screening pages & invitations: canada.ca

7. Saskatchewan Cancer Agency — Screening programs (BreastCheck, CervixCheck, ColonCheck): saskcancer.ca

www.ingramcontent.com/pod-product-compliance
Lightning Source LLC
Chambersburg PA
CBHW040912210326
41597CB00030B/5062